D0365163

# VD
# THE ABC's

by
## John W. Grover, M.D.

Assistant Clinical Professor of Obstetrics and Gynecology,
Harvard Medical School,
and
Chief of Women's Ambulatory Clinics,
Massachusetts General Hospital

## with
## Dick Grace

and a foreword by
## Nicholas J. Fiumara, M.D.

Director, Division of Communicable and Venereal Diseases,
Massachusetts Department of Public Health

**PRENTICE-HALL, INC.**
Englewood Cliffs, New Jersey

*This book is dedicated to Jessica,
Amy, and Ava Grover and to
Doreen and Richard Grace.
We hope that it will help change
the social pressures to which
they are subjected, and help them
individually meet and deal with
these problems more effectively
than we did in our youth.*

*VD: The ABC's* by John Wagner Grover, M.D., with Dick Grace
Copyright © 1971 by John Wagner Grover, M.D., and Dick Grace
All rights reserved. No part of this book may be
reproduced in any form or by any means, except for
the inclusion of brief quotations in a review, without
permission in writing from the publisher.
ISBN 0-13-939900-3 (casebound)
    0-13-939918-6 (paperbound)
Library of Congress Catalog Card Number: 76-168623
Printed in the United States of America T
Prentice-Hall International, Inc., London
Prentice-Hall of Australia, Pty. Ltd., Sydney
Prentice-Hall of Canada, Ltd., Toronto
Prentice-Hall of India Private Ltd., New Delhi
Prentice-Hall of Japan, Inc., Tokyo

**Fourth Printing.......April, 1972**

# CONTENTS

616.951
G88

108420

# FOREWORD

GONORRHEA AND SYPHILIS continue to be major causes of concern to all who are interested in, and responsible for, the health of the community and its people. In the United States, there are about two million patients infected with gonorrhea each year, and about eighty thousand new cases of syphilis—a ratio of about twenty-five patients with gonorrhea, to one with primary or secondary syphilis. Unfortunately, a disproportionately higher percentage of infected people are teenagers. In 1970, approximately twenty-five percent of reported infectious venereal disease was in the ages ten to nineteen, and more than six out of ten patients were under twenty-five years old. Society and the medical profession have a right to be concerned about our young people. However, any discussion of the problem of venereal diseases among our youth would be relatively meaningless, unless we took into account the environment in which they live and grow.

The United States has changed from an agricultural, rural society to an urban and now suburban technocracy. Our society has become more complex. We have changed greatly from the time when the family and the extended family lived in close association: when the father worked nearby, and was in and out of the home several times daily, when children shared in maintaining the home, when recreation was family centered, when education began in the home and was closely supervised, when religious training was part of the heritage, when growing children were supervised by their parents and the adults of the extended family. We now have a sub-urbanization of the family. Father works away from home; there are more working mothers today than there are working single women; there is dispersion of family members, with only a traditional family gathering on the holidays. The extended family has also been dispersed, so that when the clan gathers at a funeral or wedding, one is apt to meet one or more relatives previously unknown. Thus, we see that the family is losing some of its historic influence for social cohesion, with more and more of the roles gradually, and even reluctantly, being assumed by other agencies of society.

As the United States advanced technically, with improvement in the standard of living, its very success created forces which had profound effects on contemporary youth. Let us begin with its impact on biologic adolescence. Adolescence is a period when a young person is supposed to mature physically, intellectually, emotionally, socially, and morally. This maturation process continues until adulthood. However, the average age at which puberty now occurs has become lower. Today, females are menstruating earlier with the average age being slightly more than twelve years; thus, they are biologically capable of assuming adult roles at a younger age. Although the adolescent is biologically capable of and interested in sex, the technical society demands that adolescence be prolonged until the teen-ager has acquired the formal training necessary to become a self-supporting adult.

For about seven to ten million young people attending college or post-graduate school, social adolescence is further extended. Lengthened because of the needs and requirements of modern technologic society, prolonged adolescence affects our youth in those very qualities in which he is supposed to mature. How has society met the dilemma with which our young people are faced? On one hand, they have the sexual capacity to act, and on the other, they must face the restraints imposed upon them.

Ours is an affluent society. While pockets of poverty exist in our country, never have so many had so much. Affluence has many advantages. However, it also has some built-in dangers. Young people brought up in a world where everything has come easily to them will face the demands of increased academic performance where rapid learning and better grades are in the student's own interest. However, intellectual endeavor is lonely work. It is tedious and does not offer immediate rewards. Freud defined maturity as "the ability to postpone gratification." Youth is bombarded with a philosophy fostering immaturity. One is conditioned to look for instant gratification. The American ideal of individual success and fulfillment through planning and hard work is being replaced by the passion for instant happiness as witnessed by the multitude of credit cards, the advertising slogans (fly now, pay later)—"Have fun now, don't worry about tomorrow." Immaturity, as evidenced by the absence of impulse control, is revealed not only in acts of sexual permissiveness, but also in aggressive and destructive acts of rebellion and crimes of violence.

Youth is also influenced by a society which fosters the philosophy of excuse replacing the philosophy of personal responsibility. How often we hear "Everyone is doing it, why shouldn't I?" "It's the 'in' thing to do . . . I don't want to be a square." There is national preoccupation with sex and a change in the social and moral climate. Inherent in our philosophy of sexual freedom is a demand for the right to determine our own modes of individual behavior. Sex is the status symbol for glamor, success, and happiness. This attitude is encouraged, kept alive, and reinforced by movies, television, and advertisements. The sexual libertarians encourage the notion that free indulgence in sex is healthy, and leads to happiness and fulfillment. Young people are told that sexual permissiveness releases them from stifling inhibitions, and will open the door to more meaningful and deeper relationships with the opposite sex. Furthermore, the new contraceptives and antibiotics free them from worry about unwanted pregnancies and disease. Those who have succumbed to this philosophy not infrequently have empty relationships, unwanted pregnancies, abortions, hasty, ill-advised marriages, disrupted careers, disillusionment and frustrations as well as VD. The offices of many psychiatrists, psychologists, and counsellors are filled with these victims.

A more modern philosophy has now invaded the high school and college scene. In essence, it states that if two people love each other, they can act as if they are married—love will make the relationship right and beautiful. They forget how many times a young person is capable of falling in love.

College students demand with increasing frequency the right to privacy and self-determination in matters of sex. The co-ed dormitory is one result of their labors. The colleges have aban-

vi

doned their roles *in loco parentis*. They have also forgotten that history has shown that the amount of sexual activity is also directly proportional to the opportunities for it. Society, too, has forgotten that the amount of sexual activity is also directly proportional to the environmental stimuli.

The sexually emancipated female fails to appreciate that the sexual act is not necessarily an act of love. Sexual intercourse can and does answer a wide variety of other psychological needs such as tension release, hate, rebellion, curiosity, contempt, hostility, dominance, submission, and inferiority.

Among high school and college students and people in general, there have always been internal and external sanctions which operate to control sexual behavior. Effective internal controls have always included conscience, self-expectation, and the desire to make sex part of a meaningful and permanent relationship. External factors included disapproval by persons important to one's self, the customs of the social group, or retaliatory loss of privileges, esteem, or financial support. Venereal disease and the fear of pregnancy have been substantially reduced because of the many medical advances of today. Paradoxically, however, many girls will not use the pill. Apart from the fact that it is a bother to take regularly, it is not considered romantic; and a girl taking the pill is often considered by her partner as always being available and prepared for action.

It is unfortunate, but true, that currently there is much about sex in America that is negative, to the despair of many. However, there are two views of every life situation, and there is much on the positive side that may also influence the evolution of sexual behavior in this country. We do have much more basic information and understanding of sexual physiology and psychology. Our new freedom allows us to communicate and teach about sexual behavior more realistically; the mass media make possible newer and more effective teaching and learning methods. Dr. Grover looks for the day when the media lives up to its full potential for teaching.

The facts about VD as presented here are true; the format of the book is youthful and media-oriented. It will be especially interesting to young people, but no matter what your age you will find the material informative, readable, and of intense and urgent importance to our whole society. The author intends the book to be used by all who are concerned with sexual and VD problems not only as a source book for facts, but as a statement of his views regarding how as a society or as individuals we can learn to make healthy and appropriate decisions. He does not intend to prescribe what you should or should not do, but rather wishes to teach you to use your mind well in deciding what you do, in place of acting impulsively in a quest for instant gratification.

Many may disagree with Dr. Grover's viewpoint, or with parts of his presentation; I do not always agree with him myself. But just as he and I freely discuss and think about our differences both publicly and privately, so should you examine carefully what it is that he says, in order to draw your own conclusions and to act upon them.

NICHOLAS J. FIUMARA, M.D., M.P.H.
*Director*
*Division of Communicable and*
*Venereal Diseases*
*Massachusetts Department of Public Health*

*PREFACE*

In the last several years I began to awaken to the immensity of the venereal disease problem in the United States. Until recently, VD was rarely experienced in my practice and in the specialty clinics of my hospital. Sure, there was a VD clinic somewhere around, but I didn't work in it. I felt insulated and secure from a problem which had become less and less important to me and to medical practice during the years of my training after World War II. After all, hadn't penicillin pretty much eliminated syphilis and gonorrhea as threats to the health of our society? Didn't the textbooks say that they were vanishing diseases? Our VD clinic became more of a clinic for medical curiosities, such as the old "lues" patient, who had been left over from past times. The congenital syphilitic, with his odd-looking teeth and other deformities was kept on tap for teaching medical students. At most, the VD clinic might receive a few active patients on referral from "outside" for further study and treatment. I recall that I personally never saw a case of primary syphilis during medical school or in my postgraduate training.

Doctors and patients alike could not be blamed for being so complacent, if the VD problem were to be no more troublesome than what we had known. But, like all things human, life never stands still, and it certainly hasn't with sexual behavior and venereal disease.

While experts argued over whether or not a sexual revolution was taking place (and still there's no agreement), I noted a gradual increase during the last several years in the number of my own patients acquiring VD. "But these are nice people," I thought. "How can this be happening?" No one seemed exempt; well-to-do, well-educated, single, poor, pregnant, married—you name it; all types of people were subject in increasing numbers to these serious diseases.

By 1970 the increased caseload so altered our care of hospital patients that I was called in distress by our clinic staff nurses. In 1969 the number of VD patients cared for in Gynecology and Urology clinics had leaped incredibly. From little or nothing, these patients now absorbed thirty to fifty percent of our time and effort, and interfered with our care of other types of patients. Even the Emergency Ward was inundated with VD. The caseload now exceeds two hundred per week, or more patients on an annual basis than were treated in the whole state of Massachusetts in 1969.

These figures sound unbelievable, but the overall situation is even more dismaying. When you break down the caseload by age groups, the most striking increase in VD is among teen-agers. In that group, cases have increased one thousand percent in five years, and this year will account for five hundred thousand cases, about one-third of the total for the United States.

With these statistics to alarm us, the question of how to prevent or deal with venereal disease in young people is clearly of utmost urgency. In making an effort to deal with the problem, I have based my views on recent and past experiences as I personally worked with young people. For at least the last five years I have participated in sex and health education programs for youth. Sometimes these activities have been related to church groups, and at other times I have worked with schools, colleges, and young parents' associations.

Aside from learning as the years have passed that things were changing in the youth culture, I came to know that though supposedly sophisticated in sexual matters, there are large gaps in their awareness of their bodies and bodily functions. This is nowhere more apparent than in relation to the present problem, the epidemic or pandemic of venereal diseases in America.

I took comfort from learning that I have a personal capacity to relate to the young people I was trying to reach. An ability to listen, talk, and explore issues came easily to me, and has developed effectively. Consequently I have gained much insight into their thoughts, motivations, insecurities, actions, and experiences.

Because I have learned so much from young people, and feel so strongly their need for honest information about sex and VD, I hope that by writing I will be able to communicate with the youth of today. I want to give them, as they struggle with their sexual development and identity crises in this permissive and stimulating society, the facts about venereal diseases. With this knowledge they may make responsible and healthy decisions about what they do with their minds and their bodies. It is for all of these reasons that Dick Grace and I have collaborated in this venture.

The book is written and illustrated in a way that will attract the attention of young people, be easily read by them, and give information not readily available in any other way. We hope that the material will be helpful and informative for parents, teachers, and all others interested in and working with this startling social problem. It is not meant to be a definitive textbook on the venereal diseases.

We wish to thank all who have made this book possible. First, my patients, the youngsters whose honesty and frankness in discussing their problems helped give me the knowledge and motivation to write. Second, I gratefully acknowledge the assistance and encouragement of Dr. Nicholas Fiumara, who has been a limitless source of information and materials, as well as an effective critic. Third, thanks are also due to Professor Thomas Fitzpatrick for reading the manuscript. Fourth, my staff has been most patient and tolerant of my irritability while I was preoccupied with writing. Ann Cousins was a model for some of the photographs, and Carole Straszheim helped translate some of my thoughts and phraseology into a younger context. Susan Klibanoff has my gratitude for her editing skills. Fifth, I wish to acknowledge my debt to my Department Chairman, Professor Howard Ulfelder, and the Administrative Staff of the Massachusetts General Hospital for their cooperation while we worked and wrote within the hospital context.

Last, Dick and I wish to thank our wives and children for their forebearance and support while we thought of nothing else but venereal disease. Now, it's your turn.

John W. Grover, M.D.

## CHAPTER 1

*WHAT'S HAPPENING OUT THERE?*

As a physician actively practicing obstetrics and gynecology in a large urban area, I draw my patients from
all age groups and all levels of society. I have progressed
from concern through astonishment to outright amazement
as I've watched the reappearance and incredibly rapid
spread of venereal diseases, particularly among young
people. Only twenty years ago these diseases were
considered essentially eliminated as personal and social
problems. Currently, in Boston, as in many other areas
of the United States, our hospitals and physicians are
swamped with acute cases. Some hospitals have reorgan-
ized the old "VD" clinics of the pre-antibiotic era. No end
to the epidemic is in sight.

Unfortunately, the treatment of the acute illness only
begins to deal with the complex personal tragedies of venereal disease. The extended effects on the total body and
the damage to one's genital and reproductive capacity,
long understood by medical professionals, seem to be ignored by sexually active people of all ages. To our griev-
ous hurt, the idea that gonorrhea (the "clap" or G.C.) is
no more than a cold in the genitals seems to hang on in
our minds.

Perhaps, if you sample with me a few conditions that I
often see, my point of view may become clear. Look over

my shoulder and you might observe with me the following situations, some clinical and some social, yet all with a common thread of disease to bind them together—venereal disease. Let's sharpen our medical insights and go through a typical week in my life and practice.

Monday, my week begins with a solid day of office patients. The first woman on my schedule is a nineteen-year-old college student who learned over the weekend that her date at the football game a week ago has a "drip" and is being treated for gonorrhea. As a contact she must be treated, even though she has no symptoms or signs as yet. She's anxious and scared and is on my doorstep early. After seeing several routine prenatal patients, a twenty-year-old soon-to-be-a-bride appears for her premarital examination. I learn she has been sexually active for several years, feels she now has a happy sexual relationship with her fiancé, but is worried about her fertility. She was treated for gonorrhea last year during an episode of pelvic pain and low-grade fever. Her fiancé doesn't know it, and she worries about whether her fallopian tubes (which carry the egg from the ovary to the uterine cavity) have been damaged. Her examination proved normal, but unfortunately, without some expensive and complicated tests I cannot give her a direct answer.

While I'm having a brief coffee break in the office, a young man speaks to me. He's one of my rare contacts with male patients (gynecologists usually are restricted to the care of females only), and he identifies himself as the fiancé of the girl I've just examined. He confesses that he, too, is worried about his fertility. He's never told her, but when he was on "R and R" (Rest and Recreation) in Saigon during his tour in Vietnam, he contracted G.C. It was a penicillin-resistant strain of the disease, but it had been effectively treated after a mild bout of prostatitis (inflam-

2

mation of the gland at the neck of the bladder in the male). During his first year back at college he had another attack a few days after a fraternity party weekend. I arrange for a semen analysis at a later date and try to be reassuring. Both persons will have routine blood tests for syphilis performed as another part of the premarital ritual.

Lunchtime arrives about thirty minutes late as usual, and just as I settle down to my diet lunch and coffee (are you still watching over my shoulder?) I am called to the operating room for consultation with a gynecology resident (the surgeon in training). Late in the morning he had started emergency surgery on a woman in her mid-twenties who came in during the night with signs of a tubal or ectopic pregnancy. At the time of surgery, he discovered instead that she suffered from chronic abscesses of the tubes and ovaries, and he now wishes my advice. Reluctantly, we decide it is in her best health interest to remove all the infected organs. This requires a total hysterectomy, a disastrous result of repeated episodes of gonorrhea.

Monday afternoon passes quickly, with no further VD encounters; at 5:00 P.M. a pregnant mother calls and goes to the Lying-In Hospital in active labor. No difficulties, just a normal baby boy pulled and pushed into screaming existence at 10:10 P.M. The delivery room nurse, in accordance with State Law, treats his eyes with a special antibacterial jelly to prevent blindness due to ophthalmia neonatorum—an infection of the eyes usually caused by gonorrhea that can be contracted during the birth process. A routine prophylactic treatment, to be sure, but it always impresses me that the state feels strongly enough about it to require that all newborns be so treated.

Tuesday dawns, and it's my day in the Satellite Prenatal Clinic our hospital runs in cooperation with the

3

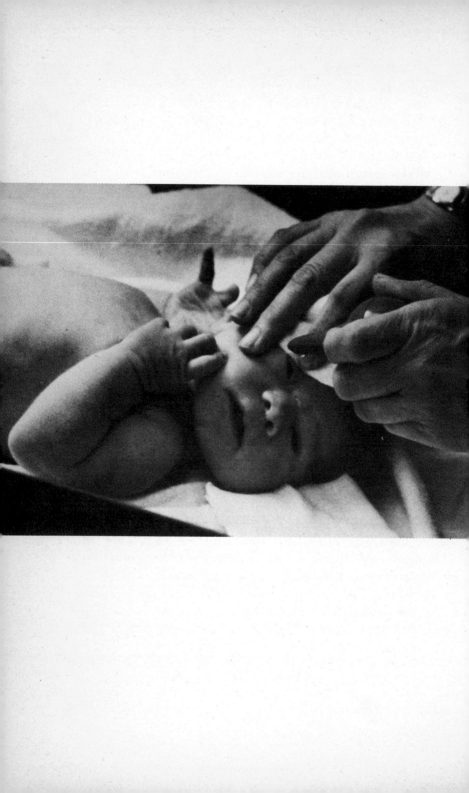

maternity hospital across town. Nothing special most of the morning except for a positive G.C. culture from a fourteen-year-old pregnant child and the hospitalization of a fifteen-year-old mother because gonorrhea complicates her use of an intrauterine contraceptive device. She's unhappy leaving school again; she lost a term when she had her baby.

Wednesday I enjoy because of the change in pace; it's my day in the operating room. Today I'm to perform the first of two operations on a young architect's wife, in an attempt to improve her fertility. Her tubes are blocked from pelvic infection due to gonorrhea several years ago. By repairing the tubes and shielding them with nonadherent plastic while they heal, some degree of normal function may be restored. However, a second major operation will be needed in six months to remove the plastic covers. Even then her chances will be only one in three of successful pregnancy.

Thursday's office hours go by easily; several patients have trichomonas vaginitis (a vaginal parasitic protozoan spread through intercourse, causing an itchy vaginal discharge), but they have no serious venereal disease. Late in the day, a call comes from a woman treated last week for G.C. Now she and her boyfriend are complaining of red, swollen, itchy, and burning genitals. A quick trip to the office shows only an acute yeast infection (moniliasis) fostered by the antibiotic treatment of the week before. A simple medication and a cream for local relief will help them both, but we all exclaimed, "What a nuisance!"

Friday is a happy day, with prenatal patients coming for their weekly check. They're all normal, so morale is high and anticipation fills the waiting room. One woman's fears about the adequacy of the treatment of her syphilis, discovered by blood tests at her first prenatal visit, dispels the mood for her. "Was it good enough? Was it soon

5

enough? Will the baby be all right?" At other times her mind dwells on where it might have come from—"Was it him? Or was it me?"

Saturday morning, I'm back again in the operating room early with a routine case and, while scrubbing my hands, have a chat with a urologist (the urologist deals specifically with the urinary tract). Seems he's about to do a repair of a urethral stricture in an older man who has had progressive difficulties in urinating during the last few years. "Even with penicillin," he says, "we still see these cases. If men only realized what the gonococcus can do."

Saturday afternoon I counsel patients. Today's patient has been unable to reach a sexual climax with her husband since he returned from a business trip last spring. Her trust in him has yet to return, even though they both were treated with penicillin for his unexpected gift of VD.

Small wonder that as I drive out Boston's Memorial Expressway toward home, past the football stadium on the way, I cringe as I hear the roar of the crowd. The radio announces the home team's winning score, and I wonder how many new cases of syphilis and gonorrhea and other assorted sundries (including pregnancy) will result from the victory celebrations and defeat commiserations that will inevitably follow the game?

My final encounter with VD this week comes as I give a ride to a long-haired young man and his rather smudgy girl. I might not have stopped if I hadn't recognized them as G.C. patients from the Free Health Clinic where I volunteer from time to time.

Of course, not all of these encounters took place in one week, and not all (but almost all) were in my own practice. I have used the clinical approach to show you some of the aspects of the venereal disease problem in our current society. VD has become a social health problem of

6

major proportions. There are many reasons: Changing sexual behavior, particularly in the young; the casual and misinformed attitudes of many who are confused, alienated, rebellious, or depressed; the general lack of interest in responsible, careful, and caring behavior of some people toward themselves and each other.

I firmly believe that the vast majority of young people (and older people, too) are not cruel at heart. They could not be so selfish as to want these things to happen. In the chapters that follow, I will discuss the broad, as well as the specific, aspects of venereal diseases as I feel they relate to human sexual behavior. I will also give you some healthy and responsible guidelines for decision-making and personal action in these complicated aspects of human nature.

This book is too short and too specialized to consider the interrelations between drugs, alcohol, venereal disease, and sex, but it must be clearly understood that they are interrelated. Special attention will be given to the situation of young people in our present culture who are pushed by peer group pressures into early sexual relationships. They are poorly prepared by their families; they are confused or ignored by their schools and churches. I do not think it wise for our society in either material or spiritual senses to allow the majority of its young people to blunder their way into maturity through these unlikely portals: premature intercourse, illegitimate pregnancy, venereal disease, abortion, and drug abuse. My bias is on the side of informed, responsible, caring behavior for people of all ages, but especially for the young, for it is they who have the most to lose and so much to gain.

## CHAPTER 2

## THE FUNDAMENTAL CRUELTY OF
## VENEREAL DISEASE: A VD DIARY

Venereal diseases are cruel infections to have and transmit. The factors that lead human beings, especially young
people, to become sexually active are so complicated and
poorly understood that the following series of case reports
will be helpful in understanding some of the pressures
that bear upon people, not only in their younger years but
at all ages. The presentation of the cases, the discussions
and viewpoints that follow, begin to tie together the nature of venereal disease. They show how we as individuals
and as a society must begin to deal responsibly with this
problem. Names and identifying details have been altered.

CASE 1

Linda is sixteen. I don't know her very well yet, since I
saw her for the first time last week; she's now six months
pregnant. Her family, probably an ordinary average
family, lives in another city, and as far as she knows
doesn't care very much about her right now. She's a
runaway, living with the street people since last fall;
finally the nets sifted her out and dropped her into our
Emergency Room late on a December night with an acute
attack of gonorrhea. Several days of penicillin shots were

followed by referral to the prenatal clinic for care during the remainder of her pregnancy. This week she was at last placed in a foster home with other runaways who have also come in "out of the cold."

She got pregnant back home and her family couldn't hack it, so she left. Her baby's father wasn't much support, either; a junkie at eighteen, and unemployed, he fled when she told him of their baby. She feels badly that since coming to Boston she has given venereal disease to a number of boys, and she doesn't know where she herself got it. For the last six weeks she's been going with Jimmy, and feels they love each other and he will marry her and help her keep her baby. He is an unemployed musician. Since meeting Jimmy, she has had intercourse with other boys, but less often than before.

## CASE 2

Charlene is nineteen years old, and has been living with Johnny for four months—or, rather, he with her, since he moved into her apartment. She has had gonorrhea several times in the past, but is ready to settle down now. She doesn't believe he's ready yet, so she's willing for him to see and have intercourse with other women until he feels ready to live with her permanently. She says he's only been with twenty or twenty-five girls and still isn't experienced enough. On direct questioning she herself admits to fifty or sixty different men, and believes this entitles her to settle down.

## CASE 3

Purvis is a sophomore at a nearby college, and I met him while on a TV panel discussing sexuality. He defines

9

promiscuity as "more than one girl in a night." He feels that sex is better in "meaningful relationships," but that it is easier for boys to move from one "meaningful relationship" to another than it is for girls. He's a youth counselor in his hometown church in a nearby suburb.

## Case 4

Elizabeth is twenty-four, and had an abortion four years ago. Since then she's been living with Charles. She's had multiple episodes of vaginitis, both of the trichomonas and monilial variety. She'd been true to Charles until this fall, when she had intercourse with another man because he was exciting and with a third man to see if he would be exciting too. He wasn't. Now she'd like Charles to learn to be exciting, since, in spite of what happened, she still really digs him. She's never had a major venereal disease.

## Case 5

Friendly is a thirty-five-year-old divorced musician. She remains on good terms with her ex-husband, an artist in another city. When he comes to town once a month, they spend the weekend together. When he goes back home, he returns to his mistress, and Friendly's lover returns to her. All was idyllic until someone—nobody admits a thing —slipped and introduced gonorrhea into this pleasant circle. Now they all have it, as well as a trichomonas infection. Treatment has involved many agonizing reappraisals of their relationships, as well as the use of specific medication.

## Case 6

Marsha is thirty-nine and married. She has never borne children, and has always suspected her husband had no sperm. As she sees the years pass, even though they have adopted two children, she remains anxious to have a baby. Because she is emotionally vulnerable, she yields to an old boyfriend while her husband is away. I'm sure she'd have been puzzled about what to do if she had become pregnant, but she didn't. She did get nonspecific urethritis, and so did her husband.

## Case 7

Emily is twelve years old. A few months ago, she was admitted to the hospital with lower abdominal pain, possibly due to appendicitis. However, her signs and symptoms were atypical, and the doctor ordered numerous laboratory studies to confirm the diagnosis. A bacterial culture grown from her vaginal secretions gave the answer: pelvic infection with peritonitis due to gonorrhea. Her boyfriend was thirteen.

## Case 8

Ethel is an unmarried mother with three children. She is pregnant again. Routine blood tests are positive for the presence of syphilis, and she must be started on an effective treatment program. She's angry with us, and insists that she has been properly treated for "bad blood" with each pregnancy. Sure enough, a few phone calls verify this. But she shouldn't be angry—she's been reinfected, and treatment again is clearly indicated.

## CASE 9

Penelope is nineteen years old. She wrote me a letter about the TV panel on venereal disease. "Thanks to you," she said, "I finally realized that I might have gonorrhea. The day after the show, I went to the nearest free health clinic where I was tested and found to have it. I am grateful to you for getting me to seek proper treatment. I want to thank you again, and so do my girl friends Mickey, Joan, Sherry, and Alice, and also Tom, Bill, Charlie, and Ed, who live with us. They are all coming in for treatment."

## CASE 10

Marie is now twenty-five, and recently I delivered her first baby. Routine you say, but something special for Marie and Don. When she was younger she'd taken awhile to settle down and had had gonorrhea several times. After marriage no babies came, and I discovered that both of her fallopian tubes had been blocked by scarring from the infections. Two major operations and two years later, Don and Marie finally had their own baby. Great! That's a happy outcome. But for every couple like Marie and Don, there are two more who fail to conceive after surgery, and others who choose not to have the operations at all, and remain childless.

## Case 11

Billie is a twenty-three-year-old single girl, described in her medical record as a practicing homosexual. She has a deprived background, and since age ten has engaged in successive homosexual relationships. She does not consider herself promiscuous. Last November she was shattered to have her relationship of several years duration end suddenly, and in a fit of depression became intoxicated in a hotel bar and was picked up by a man. Six weeks later I was asked to see her for confirmation of pregnancy. On examination, she was not only pregnant as advertised, but also had gonorrhea and trichomonas vaginitis. She was in deep despair over what was happening to her, and asked us for help. She muttered sadly as she left, "This is a helluva welcome to the heterosexual world!"

## Case 12

Eleanor is a prostitute in her twenties. I first saw her as a patient during her third pregnancy, while she was being treated for gonorrhea. After she had the baby, she tried to make a go of it with the child (her first two had been given up for adoption), but the baby died at six weeks of age from congenital heart disease unrelated to the mother's prior VD. Eleanor drifted back into prostitution in another city, became homesick and returned to Boston. She promptly picked up gonorrhea again. Because of subsequent pelvic inflammation, I removed the intrauterine contraceptive device which I had placed after the last baby. She's back at work now, but on birth-control pills. We are following her case closely hoping to keep her free

13

of VD as much as possible. The last time I saw her, she wondered if she could stay clean long enough to raise her rates.

I have given you case histories of patients I have personally treated or known about directly, so that you may see that the diseases I describe have impact and meaning in the lives of real people. In each of the above situations, there is a common undercurrent of unconcern, of not caring about the well-being of one another. To me, this is far more cruel than any of the physical conditions brought about by the venereal diseases themselves. Unconcern is one of the factors that increases the incidence of venereal disease, in spite of our new sophistication about sex.

The casualness with which many of the patients entered into sexual relationships is apparent; no more so than in the following case of Cheryl, a daughter of a colleague of mine. She's a creature of her culture; one legal abortion at age eighteen, none since because of birth-control pills. When I asked her if she was in a stable relationship now, she said, "Well, more or less. Only one or two guys." When I asked her if she had ever engaged in intercourse on first dates, she said, "Not so much any more, and then only if I like him."

In our casual society few take the time to consider whether or not to have intercourse; they just do it. Likewise, there is a hesitancy to treat disease quickly when its presence is suspected. Some young people get a perverse or macabre thrill out of purposely infecting others. Some are so ignorant of the seriousness of those infections that they tell their partners about being treated only *after* they have intercourse.

We are now beginning to see how many people are in reality affected by the cruelties of venereal disease. The discomfort and inconvenience of antibiotic treatment is

14

bad enough, even when the diagnosis is made early. The miseries of acute infection, congenital disease, and sterility are obvious and even more tragic in the course of time. But the fundamental, the basic cruelty is that these conditions are in fact preventable—but we do not care enough to try.

## CHAPTER 3

## WHAT IS VENEREAL
## DISEASE ANYWAY?

Human beings are complex higher organisms belonging to the group of animals called mammals. This classification, which includes dogs and apes as well as man, applies to warm-blooded vertebrates (animals with backbones) which give birth to living young who nurse at the mother's breast. In common with birds, but in contrast to most fishes and reptiles, mammalian reproduction requires the direct transfer of semen or sperm from the body or sex organ of the male to the body or sex organ of the female.

The sex organs of male and female mammals are partially covered or lined with moist skin or mucous membranes which come into direct and intimate contact during intercourse. Contact between these body coverings allows for the transfer of disease organisms between sex partners. Just as respiratory diseases are highly specific and infect a particular target organ, the same is true of diseases that affect the male and female reproductive organs. These diseases are so specialized that they are only contracted through warm, moist, and intimate mucosal contact, conditions well met during coitus.

There are many such diseases, and they vary from conditions that are quite mild and of nuisance value only, to serious and life-threatening illnesses that spread from the reproductive tract to the entire body. These infections

16

have been known for centuries as "venereal diseases" because of their association with the genitals and the act of love or intercourse (coitus). The word *venereal* is derived from Venus, the goddess of love; another similar term often associated with VD is "venery," the pursuit of base sexual pleasures.

The venereal diseases are as old as man himself and have been known from the earliest of times. It is possible that they evolved along with man from lower life forms that were also diseased, and matched his development step by step. However they came to be in our species, today there are several major venereal diseases of importance to human society. Their incidence has increased markedly in the last few years all over the world, with corresponding increases in illness and death. The two most serious bacterial venereal diseases are syphilis and gonorrhea. Less important infections include chancroid, lymphogranuloma venereum, and granuloma inguinale. There are minor infections, such as simple warts, cold sores, and vaginitis, plus a mild disease whose cause remains obscure, hence its name of nonspecific urethritis.

## VENEREAL DISEASE IN HUMAN HISTORY

An appropriately well-rounded understanding of VD must include consideration of the historical development of our knowledge of them, and how our attitudes have grown and changed. The remainder of this chapter presents the background of VD. Later chapters relate specific details of each disease, its diagnosis, and its treatment. Although the current VD experience is thought-provoking, if not frightening, it is not the first time these diseases have appeared and caught the people's imagination. Mention of diseases which could have been syphilis and

17

gonorrhea appear in the most ancient medical writings, including those of Hippocrates and Galen more than two thousand years ago.

Our modern awareness of syphilis as a disease begins at the time of Columbus. Sailors brought a virulent strain of the spirochete back from the West Indies to Europe at the end of the fifteenth century, and the disease swept across the continent. VD remained endemic in Europe for the next several centuries, and little new knowledge developed.

By the time of King Charles II of England (seventeenth century), during the scientific renaissance, there were grave concerns about these disease conditions. As now, it was a time of great sexual freedom and permissiveness. Concern about VD was one of the reasons for the development of penile sheaths. Made from sheep intestine, the invention is commonly attributed to a French military physician, Colonel Condom, in the service of the English King. Condoms (named after the colonel) not only helped prevent the transmission of VD, but turned out to have contraceptive effects as well. Their significance in the latter area far outweighs their contribution as prophylaxis for disease. In fact, the development of condoms opened up rational possibilities for birth control and family planning, which were to become of immense practical importance in the future. In a later chapter, the relationships between venereal disease and birth control are explored.

Medical folklore associated with the treatment of venereal diseases is as fascinating as the history of the diseases themselves. Nostrums and potions, biblical laws, witchcraft and alchemy all have taken their therapeutic turns as the centuries passed. In the early decades of this century a chemical containing arsenic (Salvarsan or

18

"606") was used with limited success in the treatment of syphilis. In spite of their ancient credentials, the venereal diseases could not be effectively treated until the development of penicillin in the 1940's.

Because sexual taboos have influenced society, particularly during the last several centuries, venereal disease remained hidden and unspeakable for an inordinately long time. As recently as the early part of this century, it was not possible to discuss or write about it publicly. It persisted as a serious health problem gnawing at the vitals of individuals and society. No one knows how many persons suffered the ravages of VD. Wars in medieval times were discontinued when too many soldiers suffered from the "French Pox"; King Henry VIII of England died of syphilis. Many a monarch and peasant alike must have had his brains addled or his water works upset by syphilis or gonorrhea.

Thoughts and communications about VD remained frozen until this century, when gradual changes in public attitudes toward sexuality and its problems opened the way for the development of effective treatments. Vestiges of old attitudes remain; many older people have difficulty in bringing these facts and ideas to the surface. One older relative in my family, when asked at a cocktail party about the subject on which I was writing replied, "My lips are sealed." With that she turned to someone else and refused to discuss the book further.

Following the introduction of penicillin and other effective antibiotics in the 1940's, the incidence of syphilis and gonorrhea dropped over the next two decades to a low point. Widespread use of drugs for VD and other infections gave promise of completely controlling or eliminating this type of disease. In the 1960's however, there was a resurgence of VD. This has been attributed to slacken-

19

ing sexual mores and increased sexual promiscuity; but contributing to the increase was a laxity or delay in seeking treatment. The emergence of penicillin-resistant strains of organisms, harder to treat effectively, is another factor responsible for the increase in gonorrhea. Syphilis, fortunately, has not as yet begun to appear in resistant forms.

## VENEREAL DISEASE TODAY

One major source of resistant G.C. infections is Southeast Asia, where prostitution and a penicillin black market (no prescription necessary) have led to unsupervised and incomplete self-treatment. Bacterial accommodation to the drug is fostered in this way, and the new disease form spreads rapidly to our young men on military duty there. Whatever your position on the war in Vietnam, it is clear our presence there has led to the transmission homewards of penicillin-resistant disease.

The frankness and openness of young people today toward sexual matters should lead everyone to a greater awareness of the true nature of the venereal disease problem. As these new and informed attitudes spread, we can hope for the reemergence of prevention of infection as a primary disease-control mechanism. Adequate and prompt treatment can help contain, but not eliminate, the present epidemic. The dramatic developments of the next few years will be interesting to us all as they unfold. Can we emerge from the present chaos with developed feelings of responsibility and *care* for one another, or must a whole generation become diseased and sterile while our society learns the hard lessons about casual sex?

In the next few chapters, I will consider in detail the diseases that we have followed through history to the present day. When the task of acquainting you with what you must know about VD is completed, we can together consider some of the ways you can help society more healthily control these ancient specters.

## CHAPTER 4

## STREET PEOPLE AMONG US:
## A DOCUMENTARY

Runaways, dropouts, and drug users are the young people who most risk venereal disease. Every city has them, all seasons of the year, and Boston is no exception. There may be as many as eight thousand "street people" in the city at any one time, and they are as rootless and unattached as the name implies. Almost every community has responded in some way to the health needs of these kids, as well as to provide for their nutrition, clothing, drug withdrawal, counselling, and other social services. Free clinics, store-front clinics, crash pads, and unscheduled drop-in centers are a few of the many ways concerned people from the clergy, medical, and allied professions attempt to meet the desperate needs of alienated young people.

In Boston, it is difficult to bring runaway and often angry and discouraged kids into a hospital situation for care. A decision was made not long ago to take care of them, if possible, wherever they might be. The Free Medical Van was born out of this idea, the brainchild of Dr. Andy Guthrie. A Massachusetts General Hospital (MGH) pediatrician, he has a special interest in adolescents and their problems. He has been heartsick over the difficulties of the teen-age runaways and drug addicts. With the backing and support of a volunteer professional staff of clergy, nurses, drivers, and doctors, and some financial support from the city, a motorized trailer was outfitted as a traveling emergency clinic. Since June, 1970, the "Medivan" has made nightly voyages into Cambridge and Boston. It contacts young people who have many different personal and medical problems, most of which would never be seen in our offices or clinics.

The original van was loaned by the Massachusetts Medical Society. Father Paul Shanley, a priest working with the street people, offered a larger vehicle, which has been in use since that September. The van is now owned by "Bridge Over Troubled Waters," an organization of people concerned about the problems of adolescents and young adults in Boston. The van has become officially associated with the MGH, and is partially funded by a grant from the Massachusetts Department of Mental Health. Medical and other supplies are donated by pharmacies, pharmaceutical houses, and the MGH. The Massachusetts Department of Public Health provides penicillin and throat culture sets.

Occasionally the van stops outside a home for runaways, and the doctors and nurses make house calls for the youngsters with runny noses, athlete's foot, upset stomachs, or just plain homesickness. Later, the van may stop in one of the busy city squares where it acts as walk-in clinic for anyone with a problem. Some of the most troubled and troubling kids are seen when it calls at an informal crash pad where kids are sleeping off the effects of drugs, or are being helped back from bad trips.

After a few months of experience, it was Andy Guthrie's observation that aside from colds, drug abuse, depression, and loneliness, the most common problems encountered were venereal diseases and unwanted or out-of-wedlock pregnancy. (See daily log at end of chapter.) Knowing of my interest in venereal disease and my work with young people, he invited me to volunteer on

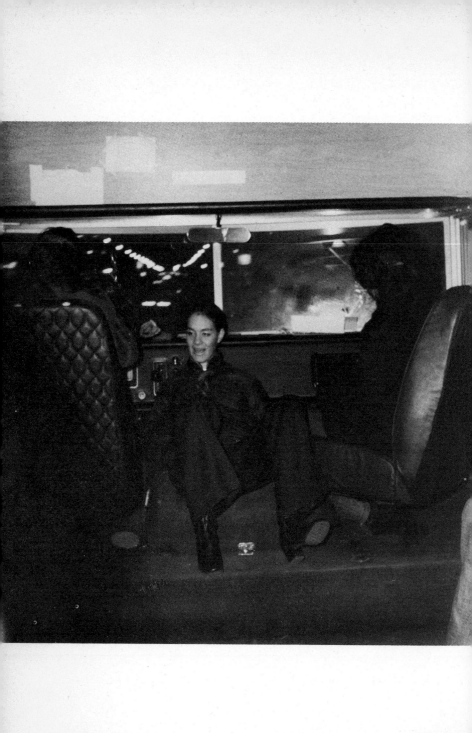

the bus to learn about this new way of delivering health care. A few nights later, I made my initial trip into the unfamiliar world of the young runaways and drug users; it was a shattering, but illuminating experience, indeed. The portion of the young I have seen in my office and heard of in the clinics represents only the top of the iceberg. The numbers of kids out there in the city who are lost and in trouble, alienated and away from home, is truly sobering. We photographed some of our experiences on that first night, and you will not soon forget what we saw.

The Medivan is an awkward, old motorized house trailer, and as we headed into the city, the winter's night was already upon us. It is bitterly cold here in mid-January, and Barbara, a young student nurse who works on the bus one night each week, is trying to stay warm next to the heater up front. The driver, Russell Jamison, and his companion Paul Bail next to Barbara have worked with young people in the city for a long time and, like the professional staff, volunteer their services to the bus. They work with "HELP," a free counselling and referral service for youngsters who need drug assistance.

Dr. John Robey, a pediatrician like Andy Guthrie, is on duty tonight; as we ride along, he fills me in on the details of the kids and their problems that we will encounter. It has been a long time since "Jock" took care of my own little girls, and it's comforting to me to know that as they have grown toward adolescence, his interest in the problems of young people has kept pace with their culture.

"John," he tells me, "you'll see all kinds of kids, some just scared and lonely and who come to see us on the van to socialize where they know they'll be accepted. Others may be sick, physically or emotionally, and some may be freaked out on drugs or stoned on pot. Most of the time we see the nuisance problems you find anywhere, like the

25

sniffles, or stitches that may have to come out, or blistered feet. We see frostbite when a kid has slept out all night, and we see a lot of malnutrition. Unsupervised youngsters eat a lot of peanut butter and soda pop.

"The kids we're going to see have a lot of trouble accepting straight people. You'll have to take off your tie and mess yourself up a little to pass muster with them. Even the nurses wear street clothes rather than uniforms."

"Jock," I said, "what do the kids think about venereal disease?"

"They don't know very much about it, John. They have little reliable information, and when they do get clap they tend to think it's nothing more than a cold in the penis and laugh it off. They often consider it is a sign of belonging to the group, and may be pleased when others find out they have it."

"But what happens when someone gets sick from it?"

"When that happens, it's usually a girl. She disappears awhile, I guess to get treated, and if she shows up again, nobody says much about it."

Our first stop was at a home for runaways, most of whom were between twelve and sixteen years old; very few were known to be drug users. They were unkempt, often unwashed, and slept in ancient rooms with makeshift furniture that was awful now, and may have never seen better days. The focus of activity most of the time was in the kitchen, since kids are always hungry, but during our visit they gathered with us near the main floor office.

Larry, a sixteen-year-old from somewhere on the West Coast, had been in Boston a few months; when the weather becomes warmer he will be on his way again. He seemed a little serious and subdued when we first talked about VD, especially when we asked to take photographs.

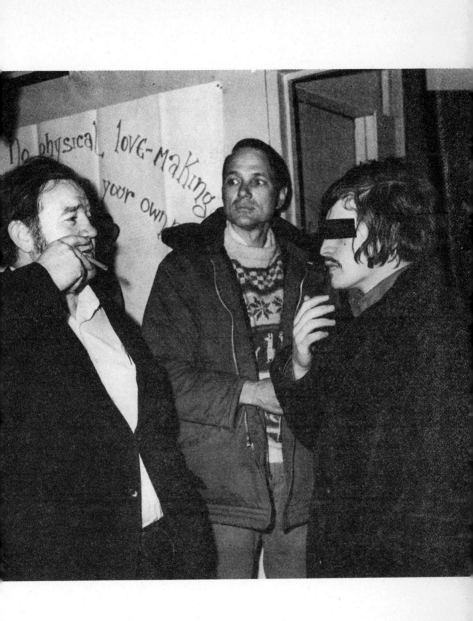

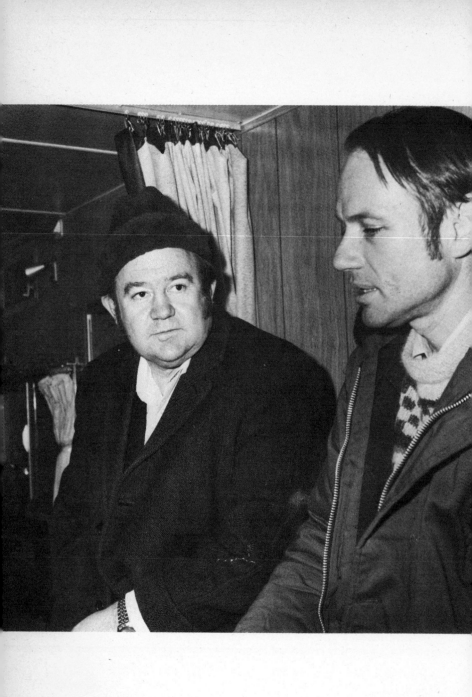

He didn't know much about VD and didn't think it was a serious problem for him.

"Larry," I said, "have you ever had the clap or given it to a girl?"

"Hell no," he laughed, "all I've ever had was the crabs!"

We laughed again as a twelve-year-old boy on the bunk bed next to me reached down and grabbed my cigar. He offered to let me play on his harmonica in exchange for the smoke. On the spur of the moment, I asked him what he knew about VD. His reply reverberated through the hallway, "You guys ain't shittin' *me*, VD is only German measles!"

Larry grew serious again as we discussed the book we were preparing. He hoped that it would help some of the kids stay out of trouble.

"Shit, Doc, you know it's going to take a helluva lot more than any book to help most of the kids." He headed upstairs.

I played my role as a Medivan doctor to the hilt, and before leaving had treated one girl with a strep throat and two with acne—it was too cold for VD!

We traveled to a square near one of the larger universities, but it was still too chilly for many people to be on the streets. One young man was given medicine for his asthma, and a cut finger that had been sewed up the night before was inspected and the dressing changed.

Before leaving, we encountered a male with gonorrhea. A thin kid, his clothing was somehow fashioned out of an American flag and clung in the cold to his drug-racked body. He wore sneakers in the dead of winter, red, white, and blue, and on his head was a purple stovepipe hat, complete with Indian feather. We gave him his first penicillin shot and a clinic referral for his dripping penis.

The nurses foraged around outside and brought back

coffee and doughnuts, and we moved on like a hospital ship on wheels.

Our next stop hit me the hardest; it was a crash pad for drug users. Inside were cots, some mats on the floor, and a few scattered tables and chairs. There must have been thirty or forty young people in the storefront rooms; some were asleep, either suffering from exhaustion or from drugs. Others were pointed out as coming back from bad acid trips and a few were stoned on grass. I didn't see any smoking or drug using on the premises. Though it looked like my bad dreams of an opium den, it was clear that here was one place where the most alienated and freaked-out kids could come for a while. They would be accepted and cared for without any questions asked.

In a corner near the window was an improvised kitchen; food sent in by a friendly restaurant owner next door was passed around. There were a few kids at card tables playing games, reading, or listening to music.

"What's in the salad?" I asked.

"Man, you wanna watch out for the avocados . . . that's where the acid is!"

At that moment I saw a familiar face across the room, and did a good old-fashioned double take. There was Linda, a sixteen-year-old pregnant girl I had recently treated for gonorrhea. We sat together and talked. She seemed happy that I was there, and introduced me to two or three of her new boyfriends.

"You remember I told you about Jimmy?" she asked. "Here he is." She introduced me to him as happily as she might have announced in another world, "and now I'd like to have you meet my fiancé. . . ." Jimmy didn't seem particularly happy to meet me. When we wanted to take some pictures of Linda, we respected the other kids' wishes and moved outside. It was still very cold.

I'm not sure whether you can tell who looks more preg-

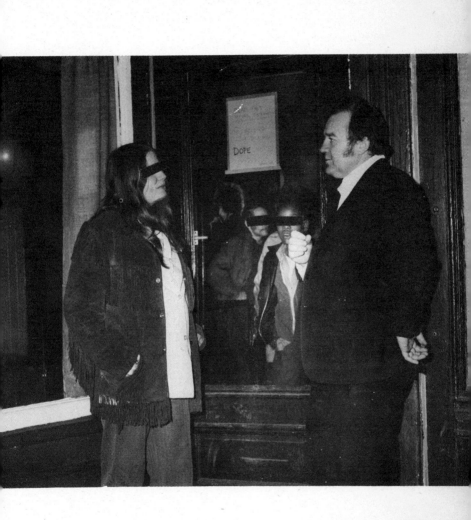

nant, Linda or me, as we chat about her baby. The interest of some of the kids in what we are doing can be seen as they peek through the door and the window curtains at us.

"Linda," I asked, "tell me again how you got gonorrhea after you were pregnant?"

"I don't really know, Dr. Grover; I got knocked-up back home, you know, by Ernie, and then when he left and I came down here, I slept with a few guys. Then I got this terrible itch, and began feelin' bad. Before I knew it, the doctors in the Emergency Ward gave me a couple of shots and told me I had it. I just don't know who gave it to me."

"Did you give it to anybody that you know of?"

"I'm sorry to say I guess I did," she lisped in her child-like frankness. "I wished I hadn't. But I haven't given it to anybody since I was treated and started to see you."

Since our meeting at the crash pad Linda has been more open and trusting with me, and I feel that the supportive relationship will help strengthen her as she has her baby. In a meaningful way, we are giving her some of the moral support and love that her parents are unable to give and she is unable to accept from them. She and her family are victims, albeit unwittingly, of cruel and unsympathetic social changes.

The van left after we photographed Linda, and we headed back across the river to our last stop. We had some passengers, since many of the kids have learned that they can get a free ride across town with us. They obviously enjoy just talking and socializing. Barbara, the student nurse, who as you can see is wearing my necktie for the evening, talks about a minor problem with one of the girl hitchhikers, and in the background Dr. Robey still wears his stethoscope. During the ride, the nurses asked me to give them the lowdown on VD. It's surprising that even professionals still don't know the facts about vene-

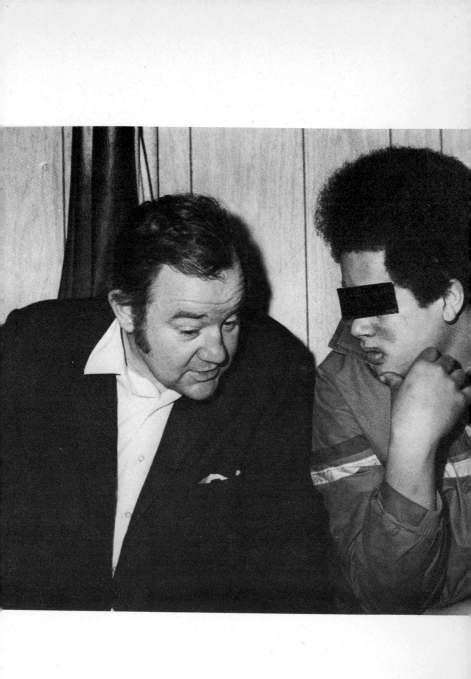

real disease, and I was glad to discuss it with them on the Medivan.

Another passenger on the van was Tony. You see us deep in conversation about a boy that I had examined a few minutes before. His belly was hurting, and all I could find physically wrong was that he was badly constipated. Emotionally, he was deeply depressed. Why? Seventeen, black, intelligent, homeless, and alienated from society. Some become radicals, some just get depressed.

Tony didn't seem to have serious problems, and like most of the kids we talked to during the evening, had never had VD, didn't know much about it, and couldn't care less.

Barbara and "Jock" finished examining a sore leg as we pulled into our last stop for the night; here we saw some of the wildest-looking of our evening patients. Long hair, buckskins, and battle jackets, unshaven and unwashed, they had the usual colds and sore feet we had seen before. As it was our last stop, and since our MGH nurse friends knew we were with the bus, they stopped by with more coffee and doughnuts and good cheer.

Close to tears, two young girls about fourteen or fifteen, both fresh runaways by their shining clean faces and clothes, come shivering into the bus. "What's the problem?" asks Paul, one of the drivers.

"We've just hit town and haven't got a pad for tonight and we're freezing our royal asses."

Paul comes out with a piece of paper, and a hastily scrawled address is passed over to the newcomers. "Three blocks up, cut over one street, and look for number 176. It'll be o.k. Just tell 'em Russell sent you. You'll get a pad for the night, but tomorrow you'll have to move on."

Robey and I debriefed ourselves as the bus headed back to its garage near the MGH. We were sobered by the evening's experiences.

34

DATE 11/30/70

PERSONNEL:
Street Worker Bob Hosond
R.N. J. Thibeault
        H. Palmer
M.D. E. De Nene
        Alex Walker
        Andy Hawkins

| NAME | LOCATION | COMPLAINT |
|---|---|---|
| 1) Mark ▓▓▓ | Old West | nausea & crush pod |
| 2) Robert ▓▓▓ | " " | Hx of seizure |
| 3) Everett ▓▓▓ | Old West | insomnia |
| 4) William ▓▓▓ | " " | Malaria x 3 yrs (URI) |
| 5) David ▓▓▓ | " " | URI |
| 6) Steve ▓▓▓ | " " | referred for counselling |
| 7) James ▓▓▓ | Place | headache |
| 8) Jackie ▓▓▓ | Holyoke | anxiety |
| 9) Edward ▓▓▓ | Holyoke | URI |
| 10) Luis ▓▓▓ | " " | ? GC |
| 11) Wayne ▓▓▓ | " " | ? GC + hepatitis |
| 12) Richard ▓▓▓ | " " | bacterial skin infection |
| 13) Paul ▓▓▓ | " " | URI |
| 14) Joe ▓▓▓ | " " | second abscess |
| 15) Paul ▓▓▓ | " " | P.E. for school |
| 16) Geoff ▓▓▓ | " " | URI |
| 17) Susan ▓▓▓ | Kenmore | ? Pregnancy |
| 18) Suze ▓▓▓ | " " | ? GC |
| 19) Susan ▓▓▓ | " " | ? pregnancy |
| 20) James ▓▓▓ | " " | ? PID |
| 21) Susan ▓▓▓ | " " | ? pregnancy |
| 22) Larry ▓▓▓ | " " | Trichomonas? |
| 23) Pete ▓▓▓ | " " | irritated (R) eye |
| 24) John ▓▓▓ | " " | Dandruff |
| 25) Anthony ▓▓▓ | " " | "Cough" |
| 26) Nancy ▓▓▓ | " " | Cold, sore throat |

One page from actual log sheet of the Medivan.

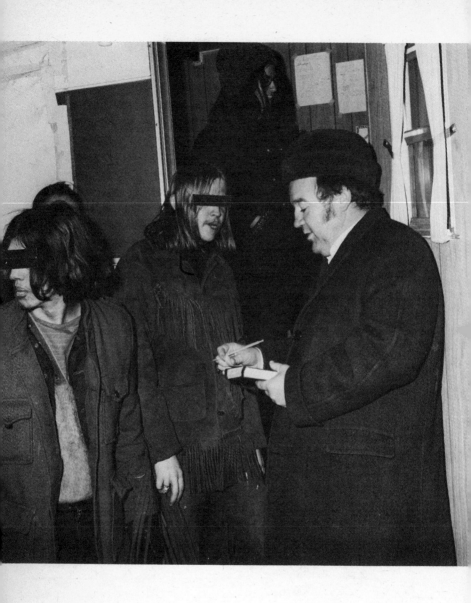

"John," he said, "people wonder what we are trying to do with the Medivan. One sure thing is we need to be there. There are a hell of a lot of kids in trouble, and I know that they can't or won't seek help for even the simplest things through the regular channels. So the Medivan came to be, and I'm on it, and I know it helps.

"Just by being willing to meet and work with them on their own terms, on their own ground, we at least can keep these kids in better health. Sometimes you establish a meaningful contact, such as you did tonight with Linda. I met Chuck Smith; I used to care for him when he was a baby . . ."

I interrupted, "I didn't hear about Chuck before; tell me about him. Did he have VD?"

"You and your one-track mind," he laughed. "No, Chuck didn't have VD. He was my patient, and I took care of him until, like you, his family moved into the suburbs. I knew Chuck ran away from home recently, but I never expected to meet him tonight. He seemed ready to talk it out, and after a good discussion of his problems, decided to call up his dad and head home tomorrow."

"It seems to me," I said, "that kind of contact doesn't occur often, not often enough. When it does, and a kid gets turned around and heads back to the world as it is, perhaps in spite of the way the world is, then the effort has been worthwhile for everybody."

37

## CHAPTER 5

*SYPHILIS—THE SLY INFECTOR*

## INTRODUCTION

Syphilis is the most serious venereal disease; in its final stages, by forming a large abscess or gumma, it attacks and destroys any organ of the body. Syphilis can cause damage to the valves of the heart and to the walls of the great blood vessels, leading to sudden death. In its most pathetic form it infects the brain and the spinal cord. In the past, when effective treatment was unavailable, painful paralysis (tabes dorsalis) and softening of the brain (general paresis) were responsible for many chronic hospital and "Insane Asylum" admissions. I remember seeing movies of syphilitic patients when I was a medical student in the 1950's. The posturings and childlike behavior they demonstrated were startling and even funny at first. That is, until I began to think about it a little more.

I call syphilis the "Thinking Man's Venereal Disease." The man or woman who is exposed to venereal disease must think carefully about it; a person must be positive that syphilis has been looked for and adequately treated. The doctor who treats venereal disease must likewise think about it, since he is the instrument by which the serious complications are prevented. Advanced syphilis has long been called by physicians "the great mimic," since the destruction of tissue can simulate other diseases, depending on which organ system is affected. For the doctor to be chagrined at missing the diagnosis in these cases is bad for his morale, but it is clearly worse for the individual patient when appropriate treatment is delayed. "Thinking Man's Venereal Disease"? Don't you forget it!

In Chapter Three I briefly touched on the fact that syphilis has been infecting man for a long time. No one knows definitely when it first appeared. It was apparently a rather mild disease prior to Columbus' voyage to the New World, but on his return his sailors may have introduced a more virulent strain of spirochete (the spiral-shaped bacterial organism that causes syphilis) into Europe. After that time serious illness flashed across the Western world like a meteor; its complications continued to afflict us for many generations. They still do.

The spirochete is fragile and sensitive. It rapidly dies outside the human body. As a consequence, infection can only be acquired by intimate physical contact, such as the touching together of the mucous membranes (the moist inner surfaces of the body) of the genital tracts (the penis and vagina). Occasionally, it is spread from the genitals to the mouth, or from mouth to mouth, if a primary chancre (the initial ulcerated lesion) is present. Like gonorrhea, it cannot be transmitted by contact with toilet seats, bathtubs, doorknobs or bed linens. Unlike gonorrhea, the organism circulates in the patient's blood for a time after the initial infection and can be spread by infected blood. This may occur when a doctor or nurse cuts a finger during surgery on an infected patient, or through a transfusion of fresh blood. Stored blood is unable to transmit the infection since the organism dies after twenty-four hours in cold storage. As will be discussed later, during pregnancy this spirochete can cross the pla-

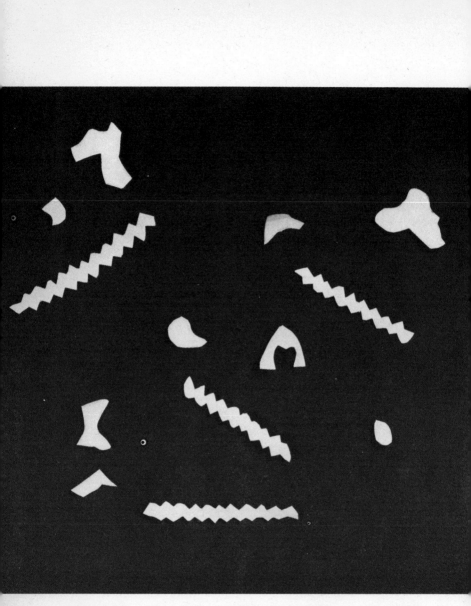

Spirochetes of syphilis, highly magnified as seen by "dark-field" illumination. They are easily identified when you look for movement and spiral shape.

centa, and infect and damage an unborn child. He will have congenital syphilis if he survives.

In this century, in this country, the incidence of cases of syphilis reached its highest level just before and during World War II. The peak incidence around 1944 reached nearly 450 cases per 100,000 population. Part of this rise was related to more accurate statistics, as the U. S. Public Health Service and the Armed Forces tightened up their reporting techniques. The strikingly rapid fall beginning at the end of the war continued until 1968. At that time the reported rate was only 10.5 cases per 100,000 population. It had reached this low level due to the use of effective antibiotic therapy. Syphilis, as most venereal diseases, is markedly under-reported by physicians. The true case incidence is much larger.

## PRIMARY SYPHILIS

The primary syphilis infection results in a painless ulcer (chancre) at the entry site. In the male this is usually obvious, as it appears at the tip of the penis. In the female the chancre may be hidden within the vagina or on the neck of the womb (cervix) and never be noticed. In either case, it is easily overlooked, since there are no symptoms. The living and motile spirochete can be seen under the microscope in direct smears from the chancre. Special "dark-field" techniques of illumination are used, and when the organism is seen a positive diagnosis can be made. The chancre heals itself within a few days, and a false sense of security may arise because the patient feels his infection has ended. Though there is no clinical evidence of infection at this time, special blood tests will detect the disease.

41

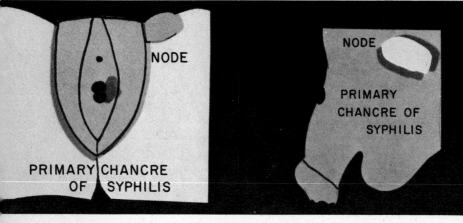

Syphilis in the female. The primary chancre, indicated here on the vulva is often overlooked. The lymph nodes in the groin are frequently enlarged and tender.

Primary syphilis in the male. The chancre may appear on the end or shaft of the penis. As in the female, lymph nodes in the groin may be enlarged and tender.

## SECONDARY SYPHILIS

During and after the presence of the chancre, the organism spreads through the body in the bloodstream. The next clinical symptoms to arise are a low-grade fever associated with a brownish-red, slightly raised skin rash. This stage is called secondary syphilis. The rash sometimes appears all over the body, and is one of the few rashes that involves the palms of the hands and the soles of the feet. Generally, itching is not a problem, and in a few days the rash disappears as quickly as it came. Unless the patient or the physician is alert, the diagnosis may again be missed at this point or confused with other transient

42

rashes such as measles or other viral infections, heat rash, or allergic dermatitis. Blood tests will continue to show the presence of the disease.

## TERTIARY SYPHILIS

After the rash is gone, the disease enters an early latent stage. The patient is entirely asymptomatic and this phase may last from a few months to four years. The next time the disease causes symptoms, however, it strips off its kid gloves and means business. It is then called tertiary syphilis. The organisms concentrate in specific areas of many different parts of the body. Wherever they congregate, they slowly and steadily destroy normal tissue. The shape of bones may be altered, liver tissue injured, and the valves of the heart distorted; the tough elastic walls of the aorta can weaken to the breaking point, leading to syphilitic aneurysms (swellings) and sudden death from heart failure or rupture of the wall of the vessel itself.

When the brain or spinal cord is affected, the patient is a victim of neurosyphilis, an especially crippling and hard to treat form of the disease. Destruction of specific areas in the spinal cord leads to partial or complete paralysis, often with painful shooting pains or paresthesias. Abnormalities of sensation and gait are characteristic. The wide-stanced way of walking, the damaged knee and ankle joints, the bent and deformed shins, are classic landmarks of the advanced case. The mind is altered when the brain is involved; the intellect is squashed, and the person reduced to a jibbering idiot-like individual who is incapable of caring for himself. He spends his days in harmless childlike hyperactivity and requires constant custodial care. Although uncommon now, these cases were once

43

seen in significant numbers in hospitals for the mentally ill and were a major burden on facilities and staff.

## INACTIVE SYPHILIS—LATE LATENT LUES

Occasionally, no further symptoms develop after early latency. If the disease remains inactive for four or more years, the patient is said to have "late latent lues," and will have no further difficulty. He is no longer infectious, although his blood test will remain positive.

Syphilis is usually infectious only through genital or oral contact in the stage of the primary chancre or initial ulceration. It is markedly less so during the stage of the rash, and not at all in later stages. However, it can be transferred to an unborn child at any stage, and direct contact with fresh blood will cause infection at any time, except during the quiescent "late latent lues" stage.

## SUMMARY OF SYPHILIS

Treatment and other aspects of syphilis are discussed specifically in other chapters. At this time I will summarize the discussion of the disease: Syphilis is an ancient disease, spread primarily through sexual or other mucosal contact during the primary stages. It is remarkably silent initially and the diagnosis may be missed or confused with other mild conditions. It is a multifaceted disease whose later manifestations are incredibly complex and serious. Syphilis can affect an unborn child more seriously than it affects the mother. The incidence of this disease is increasing rapidly in all sectors of society, tragically so among young people.

An interesting and important sidelight to syphilis, and

44

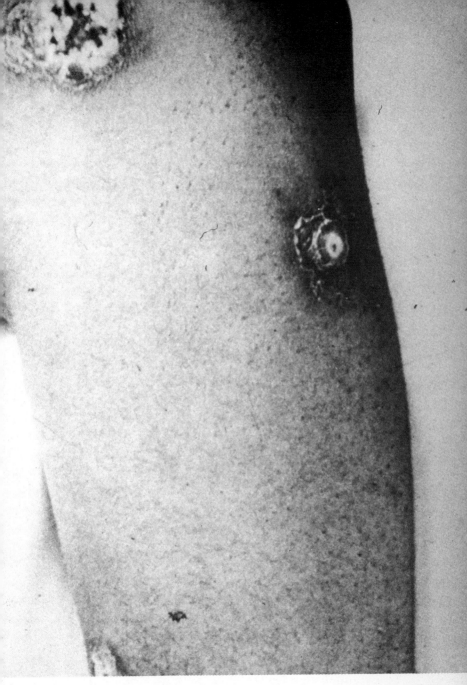

Ulcerations of secondary syphilis can appear anywhere on the body.

also to gonorrhea, is that immunity is not acquired by having either disease. Each can be contracted multiple times, and each is equally hazardous to one's health every time it is acquired. A sly, clever, and cruel infector indeed!

## OTHER SPIROCHETAL INFECTIONS

Several infectious diseases found in the tropics are caused by spirochetes and grouped with the treponemal diseases. They are not, however, venereal diseases. They have exotic names, like Yaws, Pinta, and Bejel, and are spread through breaks in the skin and mucous membranes, or through contact with the mouth and pharynx. Sexual contact may spread these infections as well. Younger people are most often infected and the diseases are usually mild.

In this modern day of rapid access to all parts of the world, more and more people with these diseases are seen and treated in temperate countries. The significance of these conditions for us is that the diseases cannot be distinguished by any known test from syphilis itself. Consequently, there are patients from time to time who will contract a non-venereal tropical spirochetal illness which clinically may resemble syphilis, yet which is not.

The identity between these tropical diseases and syphilis leads us to interesting speculations regarding the ancient origins of syphilis, which are in some contrast to the "Columbus" theory. According to the "African" theory, syphilis began as a mild, generally infectious tropical disease, spread through simple body contacts. As the disease migrated with man to temperate climates, the infective organism evolved into a more virulent form that could only be spread by direct mucosal contact. The cool

46

temperatures and dry surroundings in the temperate zones killed the organisms quickly when they were outside the body.

No matter how syphilis originated in man, we need to squarely face the challenge it offers us today. We must strive to control and ultimately eliminate this cruel and vicious disease. We must recognize that the prevention and control of syphilis begins with you and me—not with anyone else.

## CHAPTER 6

## GONORRHEA—THE FRIENDLY STERILIZER

### INTRODUCTION

Gonorrhea is more prevalent today than is syphilis; twenty times as many cases of gonorrhea are reported. Because its effects on the body are usually more limited than those of syphilis, it is considered second in importance. However, do not be deceived by its lower ranking.

In 1968 there were nearly 450,000 cases of gonorrhea reported in the United States, and there has been a sharp increase in each succeeding year. The cases reported since 1960 have more than quadrupled, with a major portion of that increase occurring in young people. In Massachusetts, and in other states where there are densely populated urban communities with many young people and students, an epidemic situation exists. There are places in the United States where one out of five senior high school students have gonorrhea. In most parts of the country, treatment facilities, the local doctors, and the hospitals alike are overtaxed and unable to deal with the great increases in people needing treatment. Special VD clinics are being organized to make access to treatment easier and more effective. Free clinics serving the street people find G.C. second only to drug overdosage as the major patient problem. At rock music festivals gonorrhea spreads through the patrons like a brush fire. It is mandatory to examine the nature of this disease carefully, in order to understand why the epidemic has come about, how it can be combatted, and why I call it "The Friendly Sterilizer."

Gonorrhea, like syphilis, has a long history. It was known to the ancients, named by Galen, and is described in the Old Testament of the Bible. One fascinating historical tale has it that at the time Columbus' sailors picked up a virulent strain of syphilis from the native American Indians, they were transmitting gonorrhea to them in return. An increase in incidence in the sixteenth and seventeenth centuries led to the development of the condom as a means of preventing infectious contact. The number of cases reported in the United States climbed sharply (along with syphilis) just prior to World War II, and similarly declined with the advent of antibiotic treatment. However, now it has become more prevalent than syphilis, partly due to the current casual disregard of gonorrhea as a serious problem by those who risk the disease. Also, the causal agent has become increasingly resistant to penicillin therapy. One of the negative spin-off effects of the Indochina War has been the introduction of these resistant strains of gonorrhea into the United States as veterans return from that part of the world.

The infectious agent that causes gonorrhea is a bacterium, the gonococcus, or by its medical name, *Neisseria gonorrhoeae*. It is a tiny bean-shaped structure which appears in pairs and is one of a family of organisms that may infect other parts of the body. (Some strains may cause no clinical problems during a saprophytic or cooperative relationship with a human host.) This organism is quickly destroyed outside the body and is specialized to the point of requiring transfer between hosts via the mucous membranes of the genitals, mouth, or rectum. It cannot be transferred through breaks in the skin or through cuts; it is not transferred across the placenta, and except in very rare instances, cannot be contracted through contact with blood. It is not as infectious as syphilis, and not every contact results in transfer of the disease.

## GONORRHEA IN THE MALE

The early effects of gonorrhea are more apparent than those of syphilis, particularly in the male. Characteristically, three days to two weeks after an infectious contact, the male will develop burning and frequency of urination, followed by a pus-like discharge that can be evoked by "stripping down" the penis. Since it almost universally occurs, most males are quickly aware that something is wrong; and often they seek treatment at this time. It is debatable whether a carrier state (infectious, but asymptomatic) exists in the male; if there is such a stage of infection, it is rare and not of much clinical importance. If untreated, the primary disease spreads locally to the upper reproductive tract structures. The prostate gland at the base of the bladder, the seminal vesicles nearby, and the epididymis (near the testicle) may become acutely inflamed and painful. Abscesses may form and require drainage or may drain spontaneously through either the urethra or rectum. Ultimately these may lead to chronic urethral strictures, and male sterility.

In about three percent of cases, it is also possible for the organisms to spread to the joints and the joint spaces, causing infectious gonococcal arthritis. Uncommonly, it reaches the heart and blood vessels or the coverings of the brain and spinal cord. These latter infections are quite rare, but must be considered as possible diagnoses when symptoms are obscure.

50

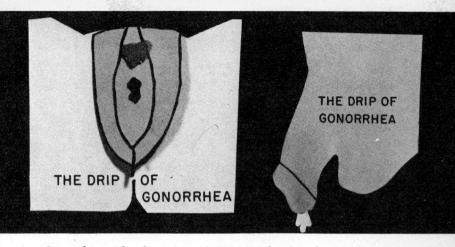

THE DRIP OF GONORRHEA

THE DRIP OF GONORRHEA

Gonorrhea: The first sign of G.C. in the female may be an itchy vaginitis and a "drip" from the urethra.

Gonorrhea in the male. The first sign is a "drip" from the end of the penis. It may be painful to urinate.

## GONORRHEA IN THE FEMALE

Gonorrhea in the female presents a varied picture. The onset of symptoms can be acute, with a pus-like discharge from the urethra and vagina associated with urinary frequency and dysuria or burning. Just as commonly, the female remains asymptomatic after her initial contact and is infectious, although she may be unaware that she has the disease. This carrier state is usually transitory, lasting an unpredictable length of time and eventually evolving into an acute infection. We do not know why this delay occurs, but it is probably related to the relatively low virulence (harmfulness) of the organism and to cyclic tissue changes of the menstrual cycle.

51

The acute infection in the female is generally localized at first, as in the male, and moves later to the upper reproductive tract by contiguous spread via the mucosal surfaces themselves. Once it attains the level of the uterus, it spreads rapidly to the fallopian tubes and to the ovaries, and a condition known as acute pelvic infammatory disease (P.I.D.) results. This causes a mild superficial inflammation of the pelvic structures, and is associated with pelvic pain and high fevers. The initial infection often quickly involves the abdominal cavity, causing a mild peritonitis which may be confused with gastrointestinal disease, and often simulates appendicitis. If untreated, the diffuse infection tends to localize, and abscesses can form which may drain spontaneously through the vagina or rectum. Occasionally these advanced infections are life threatening, as when a large tubo-ovarian abscess ruptures into the abdominal cavity and poisonous effects then cause rapid shock and death.

## "THE FRIENDLY STERILIZER"

More commonly the diagnosis is made early and proper treatment instituted. If the female is treated early, as the result of being a reported G.C. contact, or during the local stages of the disease, it is likely that there is no permanent damage to fertility. However, once the infection reaches the tubes and ovaries, the inflammatory reaction, no matter how quickly treated, results in scarring and fibrosis that distorts the anatomy of the tubes; the ovum cannot then be transported from the ovary to the uterus. This kind of sterility is hard to treat with success, and may require major surgery for correction.

Infertility specialists now describe the aftereffects of gonorrhea as the leading preventable cause of sterility in

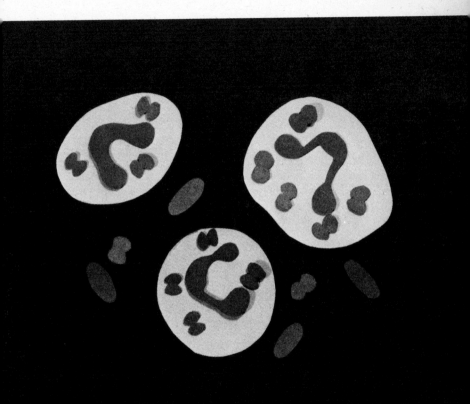

Gonorrhea

A diagram of a Gram stained smear of pus from the urethra. The large cells are white cells or pus cells, and the bean-shaped pairs of organisms within the cells are gonococci.

women. The proportion will inevitably increase as the long-term results of the current pandemic become evident. Many young people describe intercourse as "a friendly thing to do" and often experience sex casually, on first encounters, or in groups where spread of G.C. is incredibly fast. I have come to call it "the friendly sterilizer." The gonococcus may well become an inadvertent birth-control method, sterilizing many people in the younger generation, who might otherwise produce out-of-wedlock, or unplanned and unwanted pregnancies. Repeated pelvic infections add insult to injury, and predispose the female reproductive tract to infection from other organisms which may be more damaging than the gonococcus. Chronic advanced infection often leads to the necessity for surgical procedures such as hysterectomy and the removal of the infected tubes and ovaries for a permanent cure. "FRIENDLY STERILIZER," indeed!"

The infection rarely may spread to the joint spaces, to the heart, and to the central nervous stystem. Unlike the spirochete of syphilis, the gonococcus does not cross the placenta to the unborn child. It is transmitted to the baby during birth by direct contact with the eyes or other mucous membranes of the infant. Infection in the eyes can cause blindness by scarring and fibrosis. G.C. vulvovaginitis can also occur in the newborn but is easily treated and does not lead to female sterility.

Syphilis and gonorrhea can infect a person simultaneously; in fact, at one time many years go, it was thought that the different conditions were manifestations of the same disease at different stages. Later demonstration by bacteriologists of the specific organisms responsible for each infection proved they were indeed separate.

There are two atypical modes of transmission of the major venereal diseases. The first of these is rape, which, though more rare than intercourse between consenting adults, occurs frequently enough to be an acute problem for our society. Every victim of rape has a much increased risk of contracting syphilis or gonorrhea. The rapist is usually a disturbed person whose antisocial behavior most likely has led him to prior venereal disease contacts. His current victim may become infected as a result of the attack. The rape victim should seek immediate medical care in spite of anxiety and embarrassment over the event. The physician must treat for G.C. as if it were present, and perform follow-up tests to rule out syphilis.

The second atypical mode of transmission of venereal disease is between homosexual partners. The male homosexual may have syphilis or gonorrhea and spread it through oral or rectal sexual contact. It is as easily treated in the homosexual patient as in any other, but unfortunately, our social attitudes are such that homosexuals are reluctant to seek medical care, especially when discovery of their problematic sexual behavior may result. Thus an ongoing human reservoir of unknown size for venereal disease among homosexuals is perpetuated; it tends to spill over from the "gay" to the "straight" world when an individual experiences contact with both sexes. This mechanism of disease transmission is not as romantic to most of us as heterosexual intercourse, but it does occur, and is an important part of the venereal disease problem.

As you can see, gonorrhea differs from syphilis. It is basically a simpler disease, which initially causes local effects with clear-cut symptoms, especially in the male. The female may temporarily be a carrier, but soon develops localized pelvic infection. Both sexes can have advanced local disease. Both are subject to later distant spread of the infection. The female alone is subject to pelvic inflammation and peritonitis. It is she who usually becomes sterile, often after what appeared to be a relatively benign infection. A rather harsh penalty is exacted by nature for what started out as a friendly involvement between two young people living in a sexually permissive and casual society.

## CHAPTER 7

## LESS COMMON VENEREAL DISEASES

As the world's population density increases yearly, and greater numbers of people become world travelers, venereal diseases other than syphilis and gonorrhea are more frequently encountered in this country. They have long been prevalent in tropical and subtropical parts of the earth. Infections acquired in the tropics return to the United States in sufficient numbers to require our brief description. The non-venereal treponemal diseases which occur in tropical areas and resemble syphilis are not discussed here.

## CHANCROID

Known as "soft chancre," this tropical venereal disease is caused by a bacterial infection with an organism called Ducrey's bacillus (*Hemophilus ducreyi*). It is primarily a localized genital ulceration, and is more often seen in men than women. The incubation period is short, one to five days, after which a small inflamed pimple appears at the site of infection. When this ruptures, painful ulceration of one or more areas on the genitals occurs. The ulcers can sometimes be so large and destructive that the entire external genitals are destroyed. The lymph nodes in the

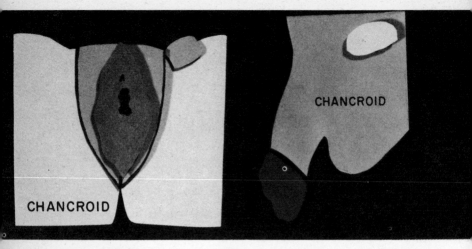

CHANCROID

CHANCROID

Chancroid: May involve all the genital organs, with inflammation of the lymph nodes as well.

groin become swollen; they break down and drain pus through the skin.

Diagnosis is primarily made by microscopic examination of tissues taken from the edge of an ulcer. The organism can occasionally be identified by stained smears from pus aspirated from lymph nodes, or by culture. However, smears and cultures are not very accurate, and the diagnosis is usually made on clinical evidence. There are no blood tests specified for chancroid.

Antibiotics offer the best treatment. The sulpha drugs and streptomycin are preferred; the tetracyclines are also effective. Drainage of pus-filled lymph nodes may be necessary, but local use of lotions and creams is unwise. Syphilis may occur concurrently, and must be searched for by microscopy and blood tests.

The prognosis is good if treatment is early and curative;

58

when the disease is advanced, the infection may still be cured, but the damage to tissues and organs is irreversible.

## LYMPHOGRANULOMA VENEREUM

This common tropical venereal disease is caused by an organism which resembles both viruses and bacteria. It is assigned to the Bedsonia group of organisms which cause "Parrot Fever" (a febrile illness in man and birds), venereal disease, and trachoma (an infectious blindness common in the tropics).

The incubation period is from several days to six weeks. A small ulcer which quickly heals appears on the genitals, and in women is often unnoticed. Occasionally the ulcer may involve the urethra and cause burning pain on urination. Shortly after the original lesion appears, the lymph nodes in the groin on one or both sides swell and become painful. Multiple nodes may be involved; as the disease progresses an inflammatory reaction around the nodes causes a characteristic matted appearance. The infected nodes often drain pus, and fistulae or passageways from the nodes to the skin may form. If left untreated the ulcers and inflammation gradually heal, but the damage to lymphatic drainage areas causes swelling and edema. In women there may be scarring, stricture, and fistula formation around the rectum and anus. Very late and neglected cases may be complicated by cancerous changes in the local tissues.

The diagnosis of lymphogranuloma venereum is made by special culture techniques. Fresh pus is inoculated into growing chick embryos, and the virus recovered from the embryonic cells. However this technique is cumbersome and time-consuming: more often the diagnosis is made by a positive skin test (the "Frei test") or by immunological tests on blood. As with chancroid, many times the diagnosis is based on the clinical appearance of the disease.

For treatment, sulpha drugs are recommended as a first choice; the tetracycline group is second choice. Penicillin is not effective. Far more than with chancroid, surgery plays a role in the care of these patients when strictures and fistulae need treatment.

The long-term chance for cure is good, but if marked tissue damage and lymphatic obstruction has taken place, a patient is permanently injured by this disease.

## GRANULOMA INGUINALE

Granuloma inguinale has a wider geographical distribution than the other tropical diseases. Cases are frequently reported in the southern United States. It is not particularly contagious and is commonly found in promiscuous individuals who may have other venereal diseases.

The causal organism is a bacterium named *Donavania granulomatis*; it first was described in India in 1905, when Dr. Donovan reported seeing rodlike inclusion bodies in tissue cells taken from infected patients. Growth of the organism in culture is difficult. The primary lesion of granuloma inguinale is a pimple on the genitals, thigh, or lower abdomen; subsequently it ulcerates and spreads to adjacent parts by contact. Swellings may appear in the groin. Late complications, such as stricture and fistula formation resemble those of lymphogranuloma venereum and chancroid.

The diagnosis of granuloma inguinale is easily made by finding the characteristic "Donovan Bodies" in smears, pus, or tissues from the ulcers. Cultures, skin tests, and immunological studies do not help make the diagnosis.

Treatment of this disease is most often with the tetracycline group of antibiotics. Streptomycin is a good second choice. The sulphas and penicillin are not effective. Expectation of cure is good, but relapse occasionally occurs. Severely damaged patients suffer from leg and genital swelling, and rectal strictures and fistulae.

In this age of increased mobility as well as relaxed sexual mores, no one of us, whether professional or layman, should overlook the existence of these diseases. Knowledge of them will help society to understand the vast problem of venereal disease and its effects, not only on our own people but on all our fellow passengers of "Spaceship Earth."

CHAPTER **8**

---

## *MINOR VENEREALLY TRANSMITTED CONDITIONS*

With increasing sexual contacts among people of all ages, the likelihood of contracting one of the major venereal diseases is high. The emphasis on suspecting syphilis or gonorrhea in many patients is right and proper. However, there are a number of minor genital infections and infestations, in some cases more frequently present than syphilis or gonorrhea. One could easily become oversuspicious and misread symptoms due to one of the minor diseases. This is not to say that any symptoms you may have should be attributed first to the lesser diseases, but if in the search for gonorrhea or syphilis these lesser conditions are diagnosed, a sigh of relief might be appropriate.

## TRICHOMONAS VAGINALIS

*Trichomonas vaginalis* vaginitis is the most common of all venereally transmitted conditions. It is caused by a protozoal parasite; a single-celled animal organism with a whip-like tail. *Trichomonas vaginalis* flourishes in the vaginal tract where it may be asymptomatic. More often it causes a grayish, bubbly, odorous vaginal discharge which increases premenstrually, and can be quite irritating. Occasionally it is accompanied by reddening and swelling

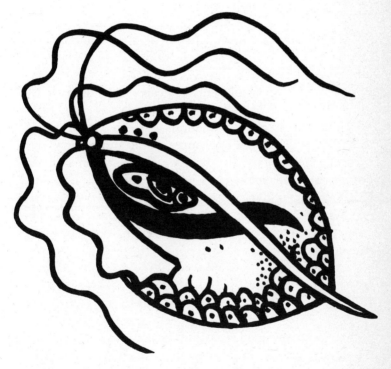

*Trichomonas vaginalis* vaginitis is the most common of all venereally transmitted conditions. It is caused by a protozoal parasite, a single-celled animal organism with a whiplike tail.

of the vaginal opening and with ulceration of the labia minora. The vagina may have a patchy ulceration which is easily recognized.

These organisms can be found in the urethra and bladder of both sexes. In the female they occasionally involve the tubes, ovaries, and pelvic structures. This results in a low-grade inflammation accompanied by dragging, nagging pelvic and lower abdominal pains. The rectum is seldom involved by this strain of the organism. The male harbors the trichomonas organism in the bladder and prostate gland asymptomatically, and consequently he is a common source of reinfection for his female consort.

The first advance in the treatment of this nuisance infection was the development of orally effective drugs; the next advance was the discovery that males are carriers. Proper treatment of both partners can easily eliminate the trichomonas organism from a given couple.

*Trichomonas vaginalis* vaginitis is treated with Metronidizole ("Flagyl") in appropriate oral and vaginal dosage for ten days for the female, and simultaneous oral dosage for the male. A single treatment course will eliminate ninety-five percent of all such infections. A second treatment at a higher dosage may be needed in some cases and a few people develop infections resistant to the drug.

## MONILIAL VAGINITIS

This infection is an irritating local disease that is seen more and more commonly since broad-spectrum antibiotic therapy favors its appearance. Certain birth-control pill preparations foster its growth. Once acquired, the fungus grows rapidly in the moist depths of the vagina

64

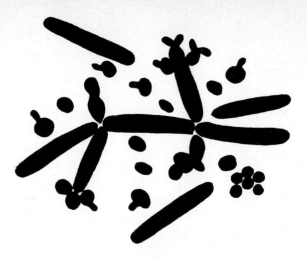

Monilia (*Candida albicans*).

and creates a curdy cottage cheeselike discharge. When it overflows onto the vulva, a beefy red, weepy, and extremely itchy and painful vulvitis results. At this stage infection can be transmitted to a sex partner who may develop balanitis—an equally irritating inflammation of the glans penis. Rarely it ascends into the urethra and prostate gland and causes prostatitis.

Treatment is difficult, largely because the organism forms spores when exposed to the air, on skin, and on clothing. Spores are extremely resistant to all forms of treatment. Cure involves appropriate local treatment with antifungal agents for at least a month, daily cleansing of the skin, boiling of underwear, and frequent changes of clothing for both partners. Often, oral antifungal agents are taken by both parties to eliminate the organism from the bowel. Douching may be indicated. Circumcision of the male may be necessary to prevent reinfection.

Diabetes mellitus (sugar in the urine) is occasionally discovered for the first time in patients suffering from monilial vaginitis. Consequently, all patients should be studied to rule out this more serious disease when simple treatments fail.

## HERPES PROGENITALIS

This viral infection in the genital tract is similar to cold sores around the mouth caused by herpes simplex virus. Herpes progenitalis can be spread to either partner by sexual contact. The painful, indolent ulceration may

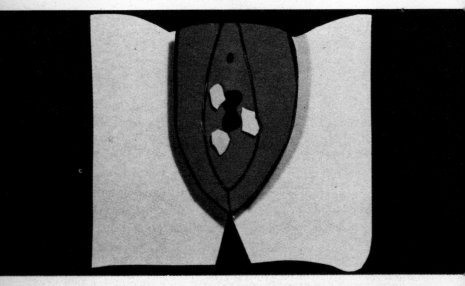

Herpes progenitalis: The ulcers of herpes infection may resemble syphilitic chancres. They are often painful and may last a long time.

easily be thought to be a more serious condition. It is often associated with one's initiation into sexual activity, or with changes in partners, and can be very distressing. In the male, the infection appears as a blistered or crusted ulceration of the glans, and may last for several weeks. In the female there is a moist, grayish ulceration of the hymen, the labia minora, and the uterine cervix. The vagina is not usually involved.

In both sexes, the initial herpes infection is painful for several weeks. Gradual healing occurs in three or four weeks. Reinfection is common, is less painful, and clears up more quickly than the initial episode.

The diagnosis of herpes infection is made by the clinical appearance of the ulcers and by the presence of virus-like bodies inside cells taken from the ulcers and studied under the microscope. Syphilis, of course, must be ruled out by blood tests and dark-field examination of wet smears from the ulcers.

There is no effective treatment for cure of herpes infections. Symptoms are often helped by lukewarm baths and astringent applications. If secondary bacterial infection occurs, antibacterial and anti-inflammatory creams may provide comfort while the infection runs its course. Sexual activity is painful and should be discontinued until healing is assured.

## VENEREAL WARTS

Wart-like fleshy excrescences that appear around the hymen and on the vulva and perineum in association with sexual activity are called venereal warts (*Condylomata acuminata*). They are thought to be virus-induced and are infectious. In the male, they occur on the head and shaft of the penis. In the female, they are associated with poor genital hygiene, and infections with other organisms are commonly seen. They can be massive and in rare cases are associated with cancerous changes. Although startling in appearance, their treatment is easy. Minor cases are treated with local applications of an anti-wart chemical, but this may be very irritating. More severe cases are

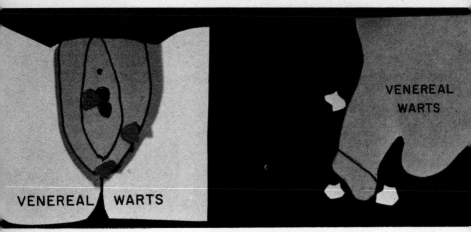

VENEREAL WARTS

VENEREAL WARTS

Venereal warts (*Condylomata acuminata*): These ugly wart-like growths are often associated with vaginitis and other infections.

Venereal warts (*Condylomata acuminata*): This benign virus-induced growth may appear anywhere on the genitalia.

treated under anesthesia either by destruction with the hot cautery, or by surgical removal. Recurrences of venereal warts are frequent.

## CRAB LICE

Although not strictly an infection, the garden-variety crab louse is transmitted through pubic hair contact, seldom through "wearing someone else's bathing suit" as is commonly stated. The infestation causes an itchy rash in the pubic area and on close inspection, the louse as well as its egg cases or "nits" can be seen near the base of the pubic hairs.

Treatment requires simple cleanliness and the use of a pharmaceutical cream containing an insecticide.

I am fascinated by our human foibles in relation to the crab louse; many of my patients calmly state that they acquired VD or pregnancy through sexual activity, but crabs—"Gee whiz, Doc, what kind of a person do you think I am?"

## SCABIES

Scabies is another itching condition that involves other parts of the body as well as the genitals. It is caused by insect infestation, and spread by sexual as well as other body contact. The tiny mite burrows just under the skin, where it is irritating. Scratching often causes ulceration and bacterial infection may further complicate the condition. As in the treatment of crab lice, local cleanliness and the application of skin lotions are needed to eradicate the mite. This condition is described by that old childhood song about the "little chigger"—"and the bump that he raises just itches like the blazes, and that's where the rub comes in."

## NONSPECIFIC URETHRITIS

Nonspecific urethritis includes a rather large wastebasket of common but obscure inflammatory conditions affecting both males and females. They are spread by sexual contact. Occasionally inflammation is severe enough to suggest acute gonorrhea, but the gonococcus cannot be detected and penicillin does not help. Most of the time the condition is mild, chronic, and tends to be recurrent, even when treated.

The male commonly notices a purulent discharge from the urethra, and complains of painful urination and discomfort at the base of the bladder due to prostatitis. The female may experience urinary pain and burning and an inflammatory vaginal discharge. The vagina and cervix, as well as the vulva and its glands, may be reddened and irritated. Upon vaginal examination, the uterus, tubes, and ovaries are mildly inflamed and tender. Rarely is a full-blown case of overt pelvic inflammatory disease (P.I.D.) thought to be a nonspecific infection.

The search for the cause has largely been unrewarding. A virus-like condition is implicated in some cases and may even cause a type of blindness in babies born to mothers with untreated infections. Fortunately, this is quite rare. The trichomonas parasite has been implicated, as it may cause low-grade pelvic symptoms. These are quickly treated with the drug "Flagyl," mentioned in an earlier part of this chapter.

The discovery of a new group of organisms called mycoplasmas is the most promising new lead in the search for the cause of nonspecific urethritis. Though they have some similarities to both bacteria and to viruses, mycoplasmas are individual enough to deserve a separate category. The culture and identification techniques are expensive, difficult, and available in only a few places in the United States. Full acceptance of mycoplasmas as the major cause of the nonspecific infection is slow. The years may verify what to many investigators now seems the answer to this puzzling infection. At this time, however, we must be understanding of a certain amount of disagreement.

Whatever the cause, most cases called nonspecific urethritis are satisfactorily treated with a five- to ten-day course of the tetracycline group of antibiotics. Penicillin is not effective. Relapse often occurs, and may be due to reinfection. The philosophy of treating both sexual partners applies here, as with other venereal diseases.

Physicians treating these patients should carry out the appropriate blood tests, smears, and cultures to rule out syphilis and gonorrhea. Once a nonspecific infection is diagnosed, both the doctor and the patient should be certain to adequately discuss the problem, in order to allay anxieties and apprehensions—whether or not any of the serious diseases were really present.

## CHAPTER 9

## BIRTH CONTROL AND VENEREAL DISEASE

### HISTORICAL BACKGROUND

One current initial reaction to the proposition that birth control and venereal disease are interrelated is to accuse "the pill" of direct responsibility for the current upswing in VD cases. It is worthwhile however to look back in time to the beginnings of our understanding of the physiology and psychology of sex, reproduction, and venereal disease for a more reasoned perspective.

Pick a point in time, several centuries ago, and any place in western Europe. The King of England is Charles II. Historically he was an amazing man who founded that great scientific body, the Royal Society, and who was a patron of the arts as well. He had some interest in another great body, a young actress named Nell Gwynne. A few years ago while in England, I had fun playing historical games by locating places where Charles and Nell had stayed together. They presided over a merry court, which was free and open about sex; the courts of other European countries of the time were as merry as those of England, and the ever-ready spirochete and gonococcus proliferated at an astounding rate.

Into this milieu came Leeuwenhoek, the Dutchman who invented the microscope and discovered sperm (his own) and described bacteria-like structures. With this new knowledge, it wasn't long until someone thought that mechanical protection between the male and female during intercourse might prevent both venereal disease and pregnancy. (The verification of the bacterial nature of disease waited until the time of Pasteur.) Thus the condom or "safe" was invented. First made out of tightly-woven linen, condoms later were prepared from a flexible pouch taken from sheep intestine. This became the world's first major advance in prophylaxis against venereal disease, and proved effective in preventing conception. We now know, of course, that VD can be transferred across oral or other mucous membranes as well as through breaks in the skin, so protection with a condom is far from complete. The mechanical view of prophylaxis persists, and our twentieth-century technology has developed the inexpensive and effective latex condom used throughout the world.

## THE CONDOM

Perhaps your parents remember snickering over the "rubbers" that could be purchased surreptitiously from vending machines in service-station rest rooms "on the other side of town," and which were inevitably stamped "for prevention of venereal disease only." When I was young these were used mostly to satisfy curiosity and provoke fantasy. Nevertheless, the devices when used reduce the transference of syphilis and gonorrhea. To the extent that "the pill" has induced a decline in the use of the condom, there is an increase in both syphilis and gonorrhea.

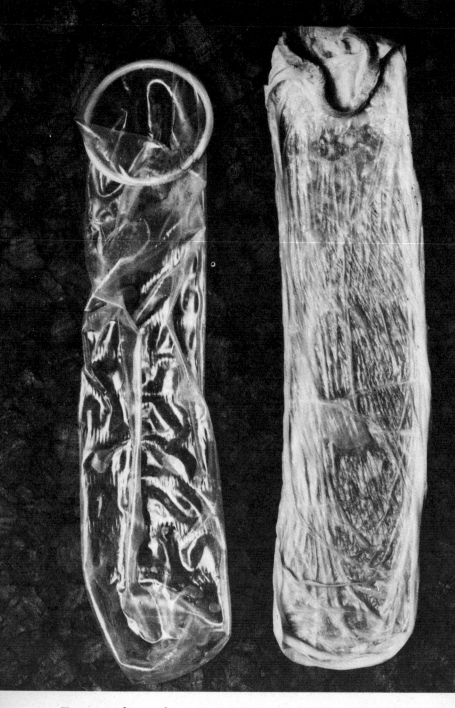

Two popular male contraceptives or condoms. The latex condom is cheap and effective, but the natural lambskin condom is often preferred. Both must be mechanically intact to be effective.

## THE DIAPHRAGM

The diaphragm is less well-known to the general public, particularly to young people. It must be fitted to the individual female by a physician. It is a direct descendant of vaginal pessaries or inserts containing chemicals and physical barriers to sperm penetration, and came into use about the same time as the condom. The modern diaphragm consists of a pliable rubber membrane held by a ring-like spring. It is placed in the vagina prior to intercourse, and when used with contraceptive jelly has a spermatocidal action. It tends to destroy the infective organisms of syphilis and gonorrhea. The VD preventive effect is not perfect. Here again, in replacing the diaphragm, "the pill" may increase the transmission of VD. By this time one should logically ask if taking birth-control pills has a direct effect on increasing the infectability of VD. There is no such increase with syphilis, but the growth of the gonorrheal organism is favored by the changes in vaginal secretions when a woman takes pills. Thus, a woman using birth-control hormones is more likely to contract G.C. when exposed to it than is a person not taking pills.

## BIRTH-CONTROL PILLS

Proponents of venereal disease control argue that "the pill" should be discontinued, while proponents of birth control feel it is an acceptable risk that must be taken. A few humorists in the professional crowd suggest that penicillin should be included in the birth-control pills to achieve both objectives. As you can see, it's not a simple and easy problem.

75

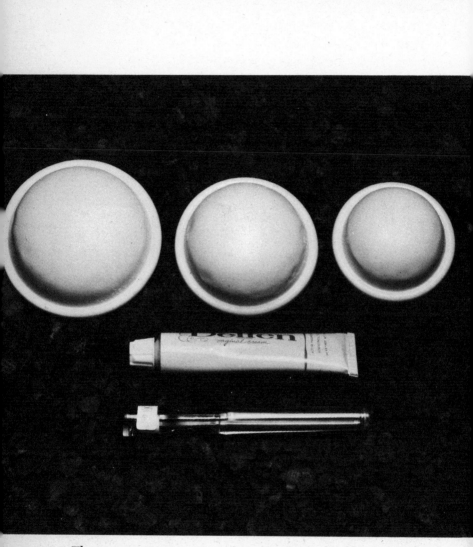

Three representative sizes of contraceptive diaphragms. They are used with a spermicidal jelly, to make them more effective. Sometimes, a plunger full of jelly is used without the diaphragm, but is less effective.

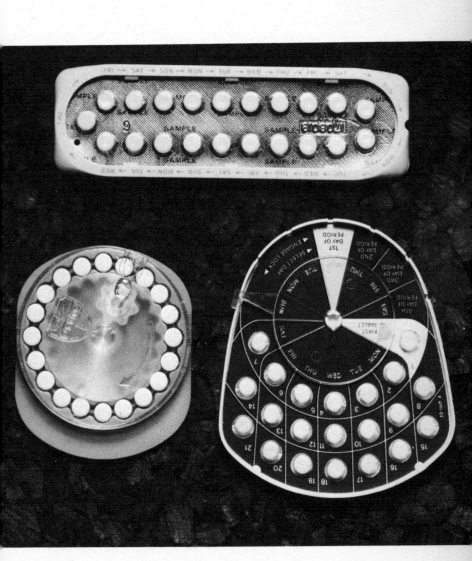

Three common varieties of birth-control pills.

## WITHDRAWAL AND RHYTHM

Incidentally, an age-old birth-control method called coitus interruptus or withdrawal of the penis at the time of ejaculation is not very effective in controlling conception. Because of the necessary mucosa-to-mucosa contacts, it is likewise not effective in preventing the transference of venereal disease. The rhythm method of birth control also fails on both counts.

## INTRAUTERINE CONTRACEPTIVES

One of the newly-popular contraceptive methods, the intrauterine contraceptive device (which also has an ancient history both in animals and man), exerts an entirely different effect on the course of venereal disease. It is

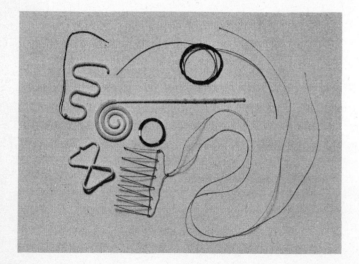

Six varieties of intrauterine contraceptive devices (IUD). They are placed inside the womb itself and stay there as long as the woman wants contraception.

made of biologically nonreactive plastic or metal that has been shaped to fit the triangular uterine cavity. It is inserted into the uterus by a physician and remains as long as the woman is content with the method. It does not alter the course of a syphilitic infection, but with gonorrhea it can be a different matter indeed. Some models of IUD's are well tolerated during an appropriately treated G.C. infection. Others, particularly those with a spring-like expansile shape, may make the initial infection more serious. They apparently allow a rapid spread of the infection to the pelvic organs, and make elimination of the disease harder. Abscess formation may be more common, and chronic infection, sterility, and later, surgery may be more often experienced.

The use of the IUD by a given patient is a decision made by herself and her doctor. If you are wearing such a device and are exposed to or contact gonorrhea, it would be in your best interests to get under medical cover fast, so that the quickest and most effective treatment can be started. Treatment can include removal of the device; this is better than risking a more serious infection. Frankness and readiness to be completely truthful with your physician is essential for good health.

## SURGICAL STERILIZATION

Surgical birth control, i.e., sterilization, which can be performed on either male or female might not be expected to alter these diseases. Syphilis, in both sexes, and gonorrhea in the male, are not affected. Gonorrhea in the sterilized female, however, is not as severe, because the fallopian tubes have been divided. One route by which the organism makes its way into the pelvic organs thus is closed. In the pre-antibiotic era, division or removal of the tubes was one way in which gynecologists attempted to arrest or limit the infection. Suffice to say, this surgery is not now a method of choice, particularly for young women who wish to preserve their childbearing capacity.

## SUMMING UP

We have seen how birth-control measures may act to prevent or enhance one's risk of becoming infected with syphilis or gonorrhea. In some situations the course of the disease may be modified. We begin to see the complexity of other problems to be faced; should we prevent pregnancy at the risk of increasing venereal disease, or the converse? This is one more area for informed and responsible decision-making. You must make these decisions if you are to grow and mature into healthy human beings during this time of public confusion and ambivalence about sex, pregnancy, and venereal disease.

## CHAPTER 10

*PREGNANCY, VENEREAL DISEASE,*
*AND BABIES*

## SYPHILIS AND PREGNANCY

The spirochete which causes syphilis circulates freely throughout the mother's body in the blood. It can cross the placenta in a pregnant woman and affect the fetus and placenta. Syphilis is such a sly infector that often the newly pregnant female does not know she has the disease. The diagnosis may be missed or delayed until the baby has already been damaged.

Because congenital syphilis is such a tragedy for a young mother, it is important that the diagnostic blood tests for syphilis be done early in pregnancy as a part of her prenatal care. The State Public Health Service requires all pregnant women to have the blood test performed; it must be done prior to the sixteenth week of pregnancy and in all patients if intrauterine damage to babies is to be prevented.

Why is it important to know early in pregnancy whether or not syphilis is present? The baby is relatively safe in spite of syphilitic infection during the first sixteen weeks of pregnancy, since the organisms do not make their way across the placenta until about that time. After sixteen weeks, however, the placenta becomes infected and its function may be so severely impaired that the

81

fetus dies and the mother has a mid-pregnancy stillbirth. Or, if the fetus does not die, it may in many ways be very unlucky indeed, since its tissues are attacked by the infection and damage to growing tissues takes place. A special inflammation around the bones and teeth is a hallmark of congenital syphilis, resulting in deformed and shortened extremities and distortion of the skull, face, and teeth. The peculiar horseshoe configuration of the teeth known as "Hutchinson's Teeth" is a lifelong sign of intrauterine damage from syphilis. When the brain is involved, severe mental retardation results; damage to the eyes may cause blindness. Infant deaths after birth are increased and fewer individuals survive to adulthood than would be expected in a healthy population.

## SYPHILIS AND THE NEWBORN

If a child born with congenital syphilis is not treated and he survives, the disease may become inactive over a period of time. The child will grow and develop although hampered by the irreversible injuries he suffered from the infection in the uterus. Once this stable state is reached, the child is noninfectious, and it is believed that such a person cannot pass the disease to the next generation. Neonatal syphilis can be discovered by blood tests as with the adult disease, and suitable antibiotic treatment given with a good expectation of cure. There would, of course, be no change in the injuries already present. The serological blood test may remain positive for the lifetime of the child, even after effective therapy.

This is congenital syphilis at its worst. However, when the mother seeks prenatal care early in pregnancy, and the diagnosis of syphilis is made either clinically or by blood test, effective treatment can be given. The treat-

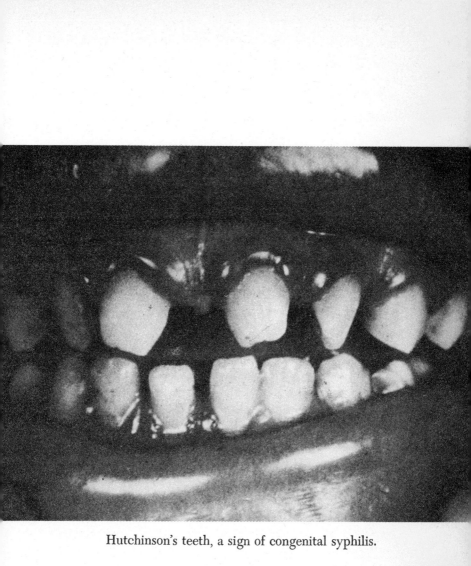

Hutchinson's teeth, a sign of congenital syphilis.

ment is the same. as for syphilis in the nonpregnant woman. Care must be taken to use an antibiotic that crosses the placenta. Penicillin is effective because it does cross the placenta, but it does not damage the growing baby. It is better if the treatment is given before the sixteenth week of pregnancy so the baby will not already be damaged or lost by miscarriage. However, treatment at any stage should be started as soon as the disease is discovered.

The patient who has once had syphilis has an increased risk of reinfection even during the same pregnancy, thus careful follow-up with repeat examinations and blood tests is mandatory. Other high risk maternity patients, such as those with other venereal diseases, should have frequent blood tests to exclude syphilis as a concomitant infection.

Another aspect of the relationship between syphilis and pregnancy is important to consider. In the patient with early latent inactive syphilis, it remains possible for the fetus to become infected. More important to the mother is that her infection may be activated, and she could develop the more damaging and lethal complications of tertiary syphilis.

Is there a relationship between a male who has syphilis and the occurrence of infection in his child? During intercourse both sperm and spirochete are transmitted to the woman; however, a resulting fertilization will not be accompanied by a direct infection in the early pregnancy. On the contrary, the disease, even though contracted at the time of the fertile intercourse, must first develop in the mother before it crosses the placenta to the unborn child. Mothers may fear that prior syphilis even when effectively treated may affect a current pregnancy. Not true. Once the infection has been eliminated and cure

84

verified by follow-up tests, there can be no delayed effect on a present or future pregnancy. Occurrence of reinfection must be guarded against. A woman's first encounter with syphilis should serve to educate her about the seriousness of the disease, and motivate her to avoid repeated infections and progressive damage to herself and to her unborn children.

## GONORRHEA AND PREGNANCY

Infection with gonorrhea during pregnancy is more common than infection with syphilis. Usually we think of gonorrhea as a sterilizing process, incompatible with pregnancy. But there always must be a first time for both intercourse and infection to occur. Thus the disease is frequently associated with pregnancy at the initiation of sexual activity, with a switch to a new partner, or as a result of rape or other unexpected intercourse. Conception may occur as well during the quiescent or asymptomatic stage of gonorrhea.

The gonococcus can at times travel via the bloodstream to the joints and other organ systems. It does not cross the placenta, so intrauterine fetal involvement does not occur. The pregnancy provides temporary protection against ascending infection, since the fallopian tubes are physiologically closed shortly after the onset of pregnancy. Transfer of the infection through the tubes to the pelvic organs is thereby prevented. Acute gonorrheal vulvovaginitis, with localized pain and discharge can occur; pelvic pain and fever is less likely than in the nonpregnant patient. Just as tubal infection precludes pregnancy by preventing transport of the egg from the ovary to the uterus, pregnancy prevents infection in the tubes by blocking upward passage of the bacterial organism. This temporary state ends when the pregnancy is terminated by abortion or delivery.

## GONORRHEA AND THE NEWBORN

What happens to the baby when the mother has gonorrhea? The infant is first exposed to direct contact with the organism in the vagina at birth; he may acquire the disease only at this time. The most serious effect of neonatal gonorrhea is an inflammatory conjunctivitis (infection around the eyes). The infection produces a condition called ophthalmia neonatorum which if not treated properly causes blindness. Because of this, all states require

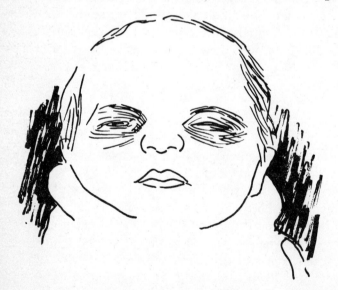

The most serious effect of neonatal gonorrhea is an inflammatory conjunctivitis (infection around the eyes). The infection produces a condition called ophthalmia neonatorum which if not treated properly causes blindness.

the eyes of newborn babies to be treated with a chemical or antibiotic preparation. This alone should indicate to any skeptics that this is a "big league" condition in our society.

In addition to infections of the eye, other mucous membranes of the newborn are vulnerable to gonorrhea. Both pharyngitis and vulvovaginitis in the female and urethritis in the male occur. In female infants the vaginal infection does not ascend into the upper reproductive tract, due to immaturity of this organ system. As with adults infected with gonorrhea, appropriate antibiotic treatment is indicated.

Joint involvement and infection of other organ systems in pregnant women can and do occur. In a patient recently under my care, the first sign of infection was acute inflammatory arthritis in the fifth month of pregnancy. Aspiration of fluid from her left elbow joint resulted in a positive smear on the Gram stain and confirmation with a positive culture. She was treated effectively and subsequently delivered a normal infant.

At the time of termination of pregnancy by abortion, miscarriage, or delivery, the patient's condition may worsen. The physical stresses involved open up blood vessels and lymph channels, and the infection spreads to the tubes and ovaries and other pelvic structures. This accounts for a small proportion of cases of puerperal sepsis or childbed fever and infected or septic abortion.

An unusual case of this nature occurred in a patient known to have heart disease who received daily doses of penicillin for protection against infection. Her pregnancy was uncomplicated, but she developed a fever immediately after delivery. Cultures unexpectedly revealed the presence of gonorrhea, and she required treatment with massive doses of penicillin. She must have developed an asymptomatic G.C. infection during the pregnancy which was penicillin-resistant, and which did not show itself clinically until delivery. The infant also was treated and remains healthy.

When gonorrhea is satisfactorily treated during pregnancy there is no reason for the mother to fear future sterility. If a flare-up of infection after delivery or abortion involves pelvic pain and fever, tubal damage and fertility problems almost inevitably result.

It is clear that both syphilis and gonorrhea are grave complications when they occur in pregnant women. Adequate treatment is available and all persons who have or are at high risk for infection must be motivated to seek effective care early in pregnancy. The ultimate goal is the *prevention* of VD.

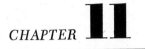

## MY DAY IN THE VD CLINIC

For many young people, the suspicion that they may have one of the venereal diseases comes as a great personal shock. It is hard for them to believe that it is true, and in many cases lack of symptoms leads to long delays in seeking proper treatment. Further delays in seeking help may arise because the boy or girl involved thinks he or she will be hurt or punished by the clinic staff or by the doctor. However, young people have every right to expect courtesy as well as good care, no matter what disease they have or how they got it. Because it is so important that you develop good attitudes toward finding medical care for yourself or someone dear to you, we are giving you this detailed description of what takes place in a VD clinic. My office nurse, Ann Cousins, modeled as the patient in the picture showing the arrival at the clinic.

The first and most important task that Ann undertook was to locate the VD clinic nearest to her. In this instance, she called the information operator at the Massachusetts General Hospital. Exactly where you call when you seek treatment will depend on your location and circumstances.

There is an appendix in the back of this book with a list of telephone numbers to call for VD information in most major cities in the United States. Or, you may call the state or municipal Department of Public Health in the city where you live. If you have access to a private physician, such as your family doctor, your old pediatrician, or a gynecologist or urologist, you can call directly for an appointment. The cost is likely to be less in a state-run or subsidized clinic, and many patients prefer the anonymity which is possible there.

Once Ann located the proper clinic, she quickly called and set up the earliest appointment she could arrange. Some clinics set aside certain times each day when no appointment is needed, and occasionally a visit to the Emergency Ward of a general hospital may be your first source of care. Most of the time, however, it is wiser to schedule your visit, which is what Ann did.

It was a dark winter's day when she arrived at MGH, and she was relieved to follow the signs to the Out-Patient Department (OPD) and get out of the cold. Once inside, she felt less anxious and easily followed the arrows to the Gynecology Clinic. There were so many people seeking help for their own problems that she didn't feel lonely, and she was reassured by a system that appeared to work well for other people.

Her first contact with the receptionist at the Gynecology Clinic was comforting; she was interviewed sympathetically, yet matter-of-factly, even when she answered the nurse's question about the purpose of her visit by saying, "I think I have a venereal disease." After a few more administrative questions regarding her address and insurance coverage, other routine matters were quickly settled. She was asked to wait in the clinic waiting room, until the changing room was available. In addition to putting on the not-so-stylish paper gown that many clinics now use, she provided a urine specimen, and routine blood tests were taken to rule out syphilis.

After what seemed like years, but was only a few

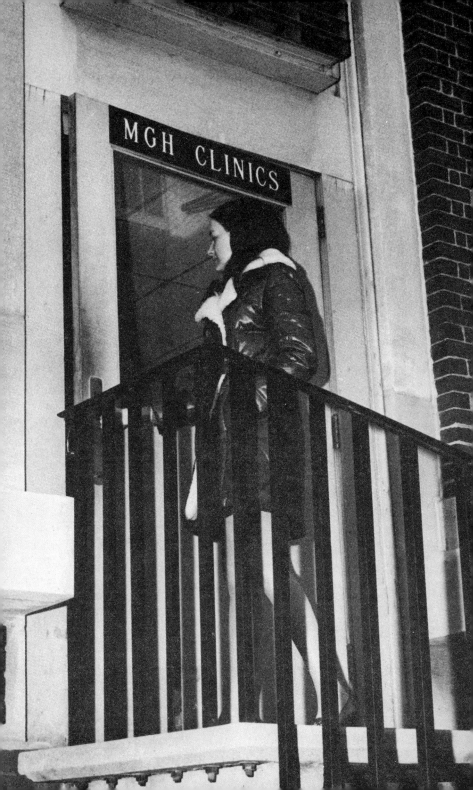

minutes, she was interviewed by a doctor. As all good doctors do, he took a brief but complete medical history for background information, and asked about the details of her exposure to venereal disease.

Sometimes, and with good reason, you may be bashful when you first discuss these intimate personal problems, but the sympathetic and relaxed air of the physician quickly puts you at ease. This is an important part of his care, since you must be frank and honest with him if you are to get the treatment needed. In some clinics, this part of the interview may be carried out by a specially trained nurse or other Public Health person who will be as expert and as comforting as the physician was for Ann.

After the interview, the doctor examined her completely to be sure of her good health, and then proceeded to perform a pelvic or "internal" examination. An actual patient volunteered to be photographed for this part of the examination, and you can see Ann carrying out her usual nursing duties. Bacterial cultures, needed to confirm the diagnosis, are taken from the neck of the womb. Cotton swabs carrying the suspected material are streaked or plated out immediately on special plates coated with culture materials that will promote the growth of the gonorrheal organism. Since this cannot be reported accurately for forty-eight hours, the doctor also prepares a Gram stained smear of the material from the neck of the womb and studies it under a microscope for the presence of bacteria. When the gonorrheal organisms are seen, the diagnosis is usually accurately made, but final confirmation waits on the report from the Bacteriology Laboratory.

If Ann had been a patient, she would have received her first shot of penicillin at the end of this visit, just as you would if you were in her place. As she leaves the clinic she has a sense of great relief, since she knows that effec-

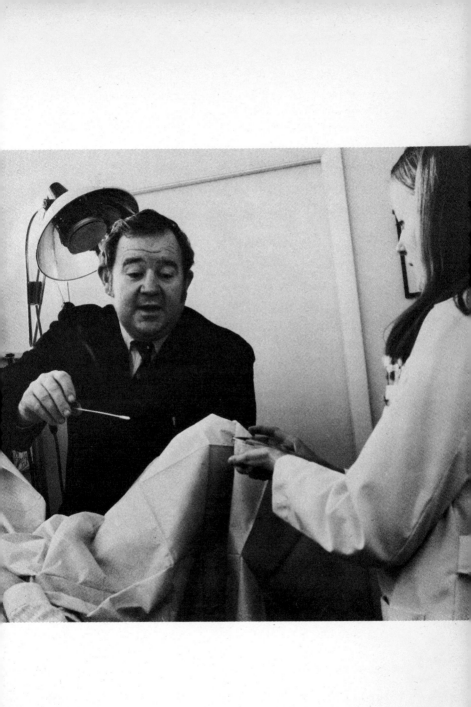

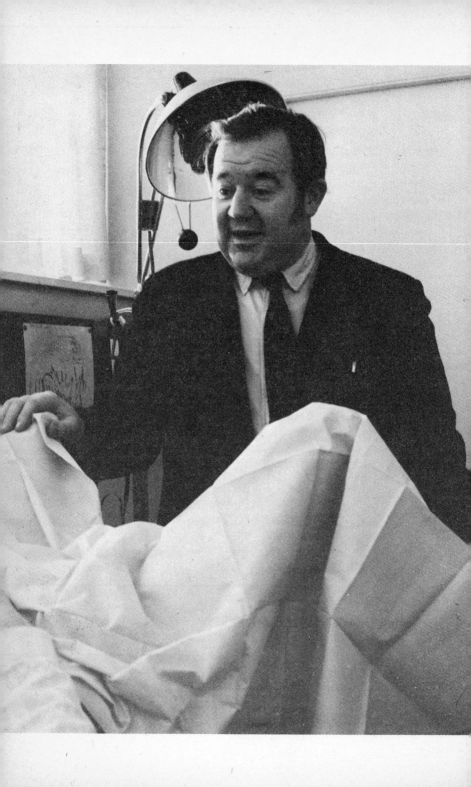

tive treatment for her illness is already underway. She is instructed to return in two days, when she will receive another shot of penicillin and learn if her culture report is positive. She also will return in four to six weeks for a repeat examination and another culture of the neck of the womb to be sure that the treatment has been completely effective.

When gonorrhea or syphilis is confirmed in anyone cared for the way we demonstrated with Ann, this result must be reported to the local Department of Public Health, in order to trace and treat all persons who have been exposed to the disease. Your privacy will be respected, and your cooperation is absolutely necessary so that the further spread of venereal disease can be stopped.

## CHAPTER 12

### DIAGNOSIS AND TREATMENT
### OF SYPHILIS AND GONORRHEA

Syphilis and gonorrhea can occur as isolated infections or exist simultaneously, and both should be searched for. In each condition, a careful medical history must be taken, in which the timing and extent of sexual contact are explored, as well as the development of symptoms and signs. The infection can then be accurately diagnosed more quickly and appropriate treatment started.

## THE DIAGNOSIS OF SYPHILIS

Syphilis screening tests: The most common method of searching for syphilis in asymptomatic patients is a simple blood test. It is routinely performed on couples about to be married, on women newly pregnant, and on most patients admitted to a hospital. Although positive returns of this blood screening test are infrequent, it is gratifying to all concerned when unsuspected cases are revealed. This blood test is commonly known as the Hinton or Wassermann test.

Diagnosis of known contacts: When a man or woman has sexual or mucosal contact with another individual with syphilis, he is considered a contact. In order to rule out infection, the Hinton test is performed. A negative re-

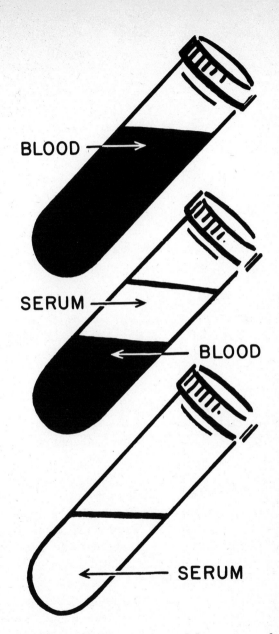

BLOOD

SERUM

BLOOD

SERUM

Preparation of blood sample for syphilis testing; the clear serum from the blood is used in these tests.

sult does not mean that the contact is not infected; a second blood test must be performed after a delay of six weeks. If the test is negative again, no treatment is necessary. If the second test is positive, treatment is indicated. In some cases the physician may wish additional tests to more specifically diagnose syphilis. Whereas the routine screening test may occasionally be falsely positive, the more complicated immunological tests are only positive when infection is or has been present, and thus may be used to clarify confusing cases. Biologically false positive Wassermann tests are relatively common, and may be due to certain febrile illnesses, viral infections, auto-immune diseases, immunizations, and occasionally to pregnancy.

Clinically infected patients: When the patient has a primary chancre of the penis, vulva, anus, or mouth, a wet smear of the exudate from the ulcer is examined microscopically under "dark-field" conditions and the living motile spirochete identified. Bacterial culture of the organism causing syphilis is not possible. By the time the chancre appears, the blood test will usually be positive, and confirms the diagnosis. More often, the positive test is the first clue to the disease, as the chancre may not be noticed.

When the rash of secondary syphilis appears, diagnosis once again depends upon the Hinton test, or more specific tests as indicated. Microscopic identification is harder to do at this time. During the subsequent latent stage the blood test is the only way to confirm the diagnosis, as in a case where the primary chancre has been missed, and the secondary rash misinterpreted or misdiagnosed.

With tertiary syphilis, in addition to the usual blood tests, spinal fluid must be studied periodically during evaluation and treatment. This allows detection of neurosyphilis as early as possible. When tissue is removed from a gumma or abscess, the spirochete can be detected micro-scopically in fixed and stained preparations.

Advanced syphilis, such as aortitis (inflammation of the walls of the large artery from the heart,) and the forms of neurosyphilis known as tabes dorsalis and general paresis can be diagnosed clearly from the history and physical examination alone; confirmation by the appropriate blood and spinal fluid tests must be obtained before treatment begins.

The blood and spinal fluid tests are necessary in observing the results of treatment; success is usually followed in time by conversion of the tests to negative. The spinal fluid, however, occasionally stays positive for years, even though the infection is adequately treated.

In any and all cases, follow-up blood tests are continued frequently for at least two years after reversion to negative, and periodically thereafter.

## THE TREATMENT OF SYPHILIS

Penicillin is the best treatment for syphilis, and in most cases an injection of a suitable dose is given every one or two days for a total of ten doses. Some physicians may give long-acting shots of penicillin, but cure is more certain when the drug is given daily. When a patient is treated for neurosyphilis the penicillin is extended to a total of twenty doses. Patients who are allergic or sensitive to penicillin may use other drugs such as tetracycline.

In pregnant patients the choice of the appropriate antibiotic must be carefully made, and treatment started as quickly as possible. In the second half of the pregnancy, the fetus may already be infected and damaged in spite of treatment, resulting in miscarriage, stillbirth, or major congenital abnormalities. An antibiotic that crosses the placenta must be chosen and the drug used must not harm the baby. Tetracycline, for instance, should not be used in pregnancy; it can be absorbed into the bones and teeth of a developing fetus where it causes minor abnormalities. Neither should erythromycin be used during pregnancy; it does not readily cross the placental barrier, and thus may not cure an infection in the fetus. When congenital syphilis (contracted from the mother via the placenta) is detected soon after birth, penicillin for the baby is again the antibiotic treatment of choice. It is given in doses appropriate for the weight of the child. The blood test in congenital syphilis may remain positive for a long period, perhaps for life, in some patients.

There is occasionally a curious but short-lived complication of treatment in patients with active syphilis; it is characterized by fever, malaise, and joint pains and sometimes by activation of ulcers and sores. Called the Herxheimer reaction, it is named for the man who originally described it. It probably is caused by the release of toxins as the organisms are destroyed by the antibiotic. Although the reaction is extreme, its effects are usually brief and harmless. It occurs only after the first injection of penicillin. The exact treatment program is best determined by a doctor or a public health team skilled in the treatment of syphilis and other venereal diseases.

## THE DIAGNOSIS OF GONORRHEA

Just as the clinical courses of syphilis and gonorrhea are markedly different, so too are the techniques of diagnosis and treatment. We have seen that syphilis is rather easily and accurately diagnosed once it is suspected. Gonorrhea, however, is harder to detect at present by our standard techniques. Often, gonorrhea must be treated prophylactically, since it is safer for the patient to be treated on suspicion alone than to risk a more severe infection because of delays for diagnostic confirmation. This sometimes confuses a patient, especially when he or she is ambivalent and uncertain both toward sexual activity and VD.

Routine screening tests for gonorrhea: These are not carried out on couples about to be married, in early pregnancy, or upon hospital admission. The only exception to this routine is the treatment of the eyes of newborns with preventive medication against blindness caused by gonorrhea. In some areas of the country, high risk patient groups such as those with prior VD or unwed mothers are screened by bacterial culture at the initiation of prenatal care. The necessity for this will increase in the future as the epidemic of VD progresses. Newer blood tests for gonorrhea are in the works, but as yet are not available for general use.

Diagnosis of contacts: When a male is reported as a G.C. contact, a specimen of prostatic and urethral secretions is obtained through prostatic massage and "stripping" a drop or two of liquid from the urethra. A bacterial culture and a Gram stained smear is made. When typical organisms are found by smear, and the diagnosis bolstered, the presence of G.C. is confirmed by a positive culture report. However, the organism is difficult to culture and may not grow even when infection is known to be present.

A male contact is always given a single course of treatment regardless of laboratory findings. It should be remembered that not all contacts will get gonorrhea when exposed. This however is no reason to avoid treatment because of a blind hope that *you* will be the lucky one who escapes VD.

Female contacts are evaluated similarly, with cultures and smears taken from the urethra and cervix. Less im-

A Gram stain smear is studied microscopically for G.C.

portance is given to a positive Gram stain, however, since other organisms from the vagina mimic the stained appearance of G.C. Just as with males a contact is given a single course of treatment.

Diagnosis of clinical infection: We mentioned in an earlier chapter that a male who has contracted gonorrhea develops symptoms in several days, and as an uncomplicated case will be clinically easy to diagnose. The same tests are carried out as with a contact and treatment is initiated. If the male is more seriously ill with abscesses and widespread disease, hospitalization for additional studies and treatment is required. Blood tests and cultures, spinal taps and aspiration of inflamed joint spaces may need to be performed to accurately evaluate the type and extent of infection.

The infected female, after a few days or weeks without symptoms, develops a gonorrheal vulvovaginitis with redness, inflammation, and an irritating urethral and vaginal discharge. Such patients are studied in the usual way with additional efforts to discover and treat trichomonas vaginalis and monilial infections that also cause vulvitis and are often associated with gonorrhea. Syphilis must also be searched for by blood tests.

The G.C. organism apparently rapidly disappears after the initial inflammatory reaction fades. Secondary infections with other organisms may occur and confuse the clinical picture even further.

Females with more advanced gonorrheal infection sometimes have a severe acute illness marked by the rapid appearance of pelvic and abdominal pain, with low-grade to moderate fever. They may appear to have acute appendicitis, ectopic or tubal pregnancy, or ruptured or twisted ovarian cysts. Emergency surgery is often performed because of the uncertain diagnosis. The true nature of the disease process is not discovered until the organs are actually visualized at the operating table.

Spread of infection to more distant organ systems in the female, as in the male, requires procedures and techniques for establishing the diagnosis. Hospitalization may be required for both diagnosis and treatment. Gonococcal infections of the throat and rectum occasionally occur as a result of homosexual activity. The search for infection in these less common locations should not be neglected.

## THE TREATMENT OF GONORRHEA

Penicillin is the mainstay of treatment for gonorrhea, even though some strains of the organism may be partially resistant to this antibiotic. Many patients fear the pain associated with penicillin injections; however, the pain is transient and soon disappears when the shots are completed. Uncomplicated gonorrhea in the male often responds completely to a single shot, but a second injection two days later may be required if symptoms

103

·persist. Two such shots on successive days are always administered to the simple proven case in the female. The more serious infections in both male and female require daily injections of massive doses of penicillin. Close observation is mandatory to be sure the treatment is effective. When fever occurs, treatment must be continued for at least two days after the temperature returns to normal.

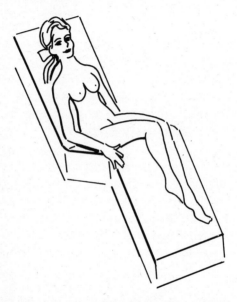

Semi-Fowler's Position keeps patient at rest in a position that confines the VD infection to the pelvis.

Both men and women, but particularly women, must be prepared for several days of physical rest and inactivity, including no sexual intercourse, if the acute infection is to be cured; otherwise a state of chronic infection is likely to develop. In order to preserve fertility, and retain her uterus, tubes, and ovaries as functioning organs, the woman who suffers a pelvic infection must make every ef-

104

fort to eliminate the infection completely. Unfortunately, this warning often falls unheeded on confused and immature ears; too often we observe the relentless progression from initial infection to chronic infection and abscess formation. Often this requires total hysterectomy. What a tragedy this is when it occurs in a young woman!

The tetracycline group of antibiotics, which can be taken by mouth, are suitable for the treatment of patients who cannot tolerate penicillin. The tetracyclines are not the first choice when penicillin can be used, since the penicillin treatment program offers the best chance for a complete cure. Occasionally other antibiotics must be used when a given therapeutic program is ineffective or incomplete.

Many patients ask why they cannot have penicillin tablets instead of the uncomfortable shots. The technical answer is that the blood levels of penicillin obtainable by oral administration are not high enough to deal effectively with the more resistant strain of gonorrhea. Since in all cases, the most desired treatment is the one which obtains the earliest and most complete cure, intramuscular penicillin must be accepted as the treatment of choice.

Young people should expect and accept from a physician a high degree of suspicion that VD is present. They should also know that the physician will do whatever is appropriate to cinch the diagnosis and plan the proper treatment. He will do blood tests or smears for syphilis, and smears and cultures for gonorrhea; he will gauge the use of penicillin or other antibiotics by the stage and course of the illness and its response to treatment.

In the final analysis, the early and accurate diagnosis and treatment of venereal disease depends very much on the patients. Young and old alike, they must willingly seek treatment. They must be frank and complete in discussions of their exposures and contacts, so that both their individual care and the health needs of society will be better served.

As an example of the wrong attitude, a girl was seen recently in the Gynecologic Clinic with an irritating vaginitis that appeared subsequent to her recent initiation into sex activity. The resident physician (house doctor) correctly suspected that she might have gonorrhea, suggested this to her, and performed the tests as outlined. Fortunately, she did not have gonorrhea, but did have a minor bacterial vaginitis which was treated with an antibacterial cream. The patient was highly agitated at the suggestion that *she* might have VD, and felt that the nurse and doctor "treated her like dirt." She wrote an indignant letter to our hospital administrator and failed to return for follow-up. Clearly, her own guilt, ignorance, and ambivalence was showing, and we wonder if she will be as lucky next time.

## WHY REPORT VD
## TO PUBLIC HEALTH AUTHORITIES?

This chapter would not be complete without a discussion of the physician's obligation to report all cases of venereal disease to the appropriate public health authority. This is the law in all states. The public health agency, once it is informed of a case, is equipped to trace contacts and insure that everyone concerned is appropriately treated. The patient's privacy is strictly protected, and certainly no civil or police actions are based on this privileged information. Without this knowledge the public health service cannot trace contacts, and the physician is less able to do so. If you have been treated by a physician, you should ask if he has made the appropriate report to

# MASSACHUSETTS DEPARTMENT OF PUBLIC HEALTH
# REPORT OF A CASE OF VENEREAL DISEASE

NAME OF PATIENT_____ AGE (OR DATE OF BIRTH)_____
(OR INITIALS OR CASE NUMBER)

STREET (IF NAME GIVEN ABOVE)_____ DATE OF DIAGNOSIS_____

SEX: ☐ MALE ☐ FEMALE

CITY OR TOWN_____ MARITAL STATUS: ☐ SINGLE ☐ MARRIED
☐ WIDOWED ☐ DIVORCED ☐ SEPARATED

OCCUPATION _____ RACE: ☐ WHITE ☐ COLORED ☐ OTHER

## SYPHILIS

☐ PRIMARY  ☐ NEURO  **POSITIVE TESTS**

☐ SECONDARY  ☐ CARDIOVASCULAR  ☐ DARKFIELD

☐ LATE  ☐ MUCOCUTANEOUS  ☐ CONGENITAL  ☐ BLOOD

☐ EARLY  ☐ OTHER  ☐ SPINAL FLUID

☐ LATENT  ☐ LATE  ☐ OTHER (SPECIFY)

## GONORRHEA  OTHER VENEREAL DISEASES

**POSITIVE TESTS**  **POSITIVE TESTS**

☐ GENITOURINARY  ☐ SMEAR  ☐ CHANCROID  ☐ DUCREY SKIN TEST

☐ EYE  ☐ CULTURE  ☐ GRANULOMA INGUINALE  ☐ SMEAR OR BIOPSY

☐ OTHER  ☐ OTHER  ☐ LYMPHOGRANULOMA VENEREUM  ☐ FREI SKIN TEST

HAS PATIENT HAD PREVIOUS TREATMENT FOR THIS INFECTION? ☐ YES ☐ NO IF YES, ☐ ADEQUATE ☐ INADEQUATE

ORDER SUPPLIES HERE  NUMBER

REPORT BLANKS _____ SIGNED _____ M. D.

LITERATURE FOR PATIENTS _____ STREET _____

LITERATURE FOR PHYSICIANS _____ CITY OR TOWN_____ DATE_____

**ALL VENEREAL DISEASE PATIENTS HAVE CONTACTS. HAVE YOU INTERVIEWED FOR CONTACTS?**

(OVER)

---

## USE THIS SIDE OF FORM TO REPORT THE FOLLOWING

CHECK ONE

☐ CONTACT

☐ PATIENT HAD POSITIVE TEST FOR SYPHILIS AND DID NOT RETURN.

☐ PATIENT PREMATURELY DISCONTINUED TREATMENT FOR_____ DATE OF LAST VISIT_____

NAME OF CONTACT OR PATIENT_____

STREET _____ AGE _____

CITY OR TOWN_____ SEX _____

OCCUPATION_____ PLACE OF EMPLOYMENT_____ MARITAL STATUS_____

FOLLOWING INFORMATION FOR CONTACTS ONLY:

CONTACT OF

☐ SYPHILIS  RELATIONSHIP TO PATIENT:

☐ PRIMARY  ☐ MARITAL ☐ FRIEND ☐ PICKUP ☐ PROSTITUTE ☐ OTHER

☐ SECONDARY

☐ EARLY LATENT  WILL YOU LOCATE AND EXAMINE THIS CONTACT? ☐ YES ☐ NO

☐ OTHER (SPECIFY)

☐ GONORRHEA  IF NOT, THE DIVISION STAFF WILL ASSIST IN LOCATING AND

☐ CHANCROID  REFERRING CONTACT FOR MEDICAL EXAMINATION.

☐ GRANULOMA INGUINALE

☐ LYMPHOGRANULOMA VENEREUM

OTHER INFORMATION HELPFUL IN LOCATING CONTACT:_____

_____

_____

**PATIENTS USUALLY HAVE SEVERAL CONTACTS.**
**PLEASE USE SEPARATE FORM FOR EACH CONTACT.**

PH-VP-13. 35M-6-65-940657

Similar VD reports as shown here are used in every state.

the public health agency, and be ready to report your contacts. Unfortunately, VD is very much under-reported, which tends to preserve the reservoir of untreated cases in the community.

Even if you are under age you should seek appropriate and effective diagnosis and treatment. In most states, the physician can legally treat you without notifying your parents or guardians. If he must let them know, you should still get care as quickly as possible. Treat your disease, and then pick up the pieces of your family life. Think how much worse it would be if your parents were not called in until you were gravely ill, in an emergency ward requiring surgery or other treatment.

Once the disease is suspected, no matter how young or old you are, get diagnosed and treated fast.

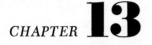

## VD AND THE CONTEMPORARY FAMILY

The differences between generations in a society where parents are too hung up to talk about sexual behavior and VD to their sophisticated offspring have led us in large part to our current impasse. Children of such parents often blunder into premature casual sexual experiences out of ignorance and unconcern. They may become alienated from their families, behaving in a fashion that actively opposes the principles and ethics of their elders.

## THE FAMILY IN THE MODERN WORLD

Some thoughtful people consider the behavior of the young as a rejection of the "establishment" created by their parents. Others see a search for love that many children find lacking because of the fragmentation of the family. National magazines examine the family in detail, and find much unhappiness. They point out, as I also believe, that in the future there will be greater variety in the ways people approach the construction and implementation of family living. The old "vertical family groups" may be replaced by the "horizontal extended family" as found in group marriages or in communes. However, for the vast

109

majority of people, the traditional family will be the mode of living together for the forseeable future.

Over the last several generations, the traditional family has become progressively limited to what some call the nuclear family consisting of the parents and their children. Today's grandparents are much less involved in child rearing; they are often enjoying healthy and independent lives of their own. Uncles and aunts and cousins are widely scattered. We are left with a hard-pressed couple that alone is responsible for the child rearing in our modern homes. For them the creation of a happy and fulfilling home atmosphere is a major challenge.

It is a *special* challenge to the nuclear family to deal with the younger generation's incredible sex and venereal disease problems. Take a tottering family that is just barely holding its own. Dad is straining at his job to excel or make the money to keep the family alive; mom's screaming her guts out because she can't stand one more day with nobody but kids. If you drop a teen-ager with VD into this family with all its hang-ups—well, you've got both a problem and a challenge.

This is where the challenge really is, boys and girls, and moms and dads. We must make this family thing work; it is all most of us will ever have. We must look hard at what it means to be a family, and use some good old-fashioned elbow grease to help it succeed.

Parents, in order to pick up this challenge, must accept that their kids look at life differently than they did or do, and must not become threatened or up tight. True, they had a generation gap with their parents, but the differences are greater now. Parents must acknowledge their kids' interest in, and awareness of, sexuality. Most parents my age know far less about sexuality and the physiology of sex than their teen-age children, and are uncomfortable with what they do know. Thus sex education for parents,

110

too, is necessary to meet the challenge of VD. They then will be better able to talk meaningfully and effectively—and lovingly—with their children. This is an evolution of family living that is greatly to be desired.

In addition, parents must learn that, in spite of anything and everything they do, how their children turn out is often beyond parental control. More and more the child becomes a product of his own culture as he grows and moves outward into the world. He is far more influenced by the media, by his peer groups, and by chance social factors in becoming an adult than was true in generations past. Parents can pass to their children ideals and ways of thinking and deciding about the issues that confront young people. They can also hope and pray that some of it will stick. An open atmosphere of love, personal responsibility, and support, espoused and lived to the best of their abilities by caring parents, is the finest family background that we can offer to our children as they face the seventies.

The challenge does not all rest with the parents. Kids, you too, have some knuckling down to these difficult problems of growing up and maturing as responsible members of your family. Try not to be afraid to involve your parents in your problems. Sure, maybe they won't understand at first. If you keep trying, most parents will show you that no one in the world loves you in quite as special a way as they do. That kind of loving relationship means that, hung up as parents are, they will try to understand and help you. There's nothing so comforting as knowing that "no matter what," your parents will support you. Your parents would like "no matter what" to include careful and responsible reflections upon what you do, especially in relation to your sexual behavior.

Here, then, is the core of the challenge that venereal disease represents. VD is a tangible focus of all of the diverse uses of human sexuality. The need for control of VD is urgent, and tragedy is near for many. One hopes that the family can rise to meet the challenge quickly and successfully.

Modern concerned families give signs of responding to the needs of their children, and I am hopeful that in the next few years there will be great changes for the better in our society. We know that when kids themselves get the facts straight, VD as well as illegitimacy and abortion occur less frequently. If parents can follow their children out of the Victorian Era which has lasted far too long, and begin effective communications with one another we will *all* emerge into a new and more mature culture.

## SEX EDUCATION BELONGS IN THE HOME

Young people need proper education concerning human sexuality and reproduction, including venereal diseases and drugs. Educating the young in these touchy areas begins, of course, at home with the preschool youngster. Attitudes toward sexuality are formed early, yet most parents of young children are ill-prepared to provide sensible and appropriate guidelines for healthy sexual development. Fortunately, books and teaching materials are available for parents to use in helping guide and educate even the nonreading toddler. Parents must also study appropriate material themselves in order to know at what level their child's interest ought to be, and in order to field questions properly.

One sensible guideline for the sex education of the preschooler is to ask the child from time to time what *he* thinks about aspects of sex and reproduction. When he asks questions, answer frankly, without hedging, and without including details that are beyond his comprehension.

112

Watching while an infant is bathed or diapered satisfies the small child's curiosity about sexual organs. His interest is normal, and should be treated naturally by the parents. More and more, young parents are free enough with their own bodies so that the toddler who is interested in swimming in the tub with mommy or daddy may do so. He will learn what people look like, and will absorb the healthy attitude that bodies are normal and not objects of shame. I realize that for cultural reasons this is not possible for all families. For those who can deal comfortably with nudity and bathing together in these important early years, such experiences can become a healthy part of growing up.

Margaret Mead has made much of the need for skin-to-skin physical contact between parents and their children. I strongly approve, and have personal and clinical observations which support this viewpoint. Recently, I noticed an example in the delivery room where an infant was put to her mother's breast for suckling at a few minutes of age. The baby was tightly wrapped, as is the usual custom, with only her face showing and the arms and legs covered and restricted. She seemed cross and mucousy, and would not nurse. I removed all blankets and wrappings from the baby and put her back on the breast with her shoulders and body touching the mother's skin directly. The mother was overjoyed to see the baby calm down and begin suckling on the nipple like a professional, though less than an hour old. The increased information the baby received from physically touching her mother gave her a better idea about what she was meant to do. I believe this same kind of frank body contact gives the very young child more confidence in his own body as it grows and develops, and is in no way threatening to the child in his early years.

Once adult development begins, this parent-child body

113

interaction is less often experienced, as the child develops a sense of individual self and a sense of privacy. At all times, parents can help in the development of healthy attitudes toward the body, as a gift to be proud of rather than hung up or up tight about.

## CHAPTER 14

## PREVENTION OF VENEREAL DISEASE: HOW WE CAN HELP

### THE PROBLEM AND THE CHALLENGE

It is often stated publicly that venereal diseases are not preventable, due to the obscurity of the initial infection, the carrier state in the female, and the unwillingness of society to recognize the nature of the problem. For instance, in many inhibited older people there is a carry-over from more remote times when VD's were not openly discussed. In contrast, many young people now feel and act casually about sex and its associated problems. Both attitudes, if left undisturbed and not redirected, can lead to further spread of these diseases, far beyond the current epidemic state.

Our present confused and chaotic feelings toward sexuality and venereal disease must inevitably change. If we remain a society unwilling and unable to deal with these perplexing and troubling situations, matters will rapidly worsen. However, if we decide to roll up our sleeves and honestly begin working toward constructive goals, healthy attitudes will yet develop.

How can we learn to prevent venereal diseases? First, both individuals and all of society must recognize that the problem exists. VD is a personal matter. It is spread from one individual, a person, to another individual. The decisions that lead to sexual intercourse are made by people, not by nameless or faceless "others." These choices relate in a very intimate way to each human involved. Of course, many do not *consciously* make these decisions, but here is one place in human experience where *not* to consciously make a decision is making a negative decision. In other words, the individual who has not made up his mind will often end up having both intercourse and VD, since the opportunity and pressure to behave this way is incredibly high at present. "Not for me," you say, "not for me. It couldn't happen to me . . . could it?"

As individuals, we must be able to make decisions about our sexual behavior that are informed and factual, not blunderingly ignorant, selfish, or romantic. We need to include the facts of VD and human sexuality in our "decision-making computer."

We should next cultivate a civilized human attitude toward making these responsible decisions, an attitude that takes both ourselves and the other person into account. We must introduce into our lives the capacity to care for one another, as well as for ourselves. Is what I'm about to do right or appropriate for me to ask of my partner? What are the ramifications of this action if I should contract or spread VD? What if pregnancy should result? Am I ready to deal with the consequences of my actions, in relation to myself, the other person (human) and to society?

Inside our skins beats a vulnerable human heart, and a complex body that is capable of great joy and fulfillment, yet susceptible to disease, and to physical and emotional pain. Stop and think a bit. The same heart that powers you, your muscles, and your brain, and the same body that gives you pleasure when loved, and pain when hurt or rejected, also exist in just as personal a way for your partner. Are we so dehumanized that we don't care any more? Are we so upset by the existence of war, disease, poverty, and pain that we do not care about ourselves or others any longer? *The capacity for making informed, responsible decisions, enabling one to act within a context of caring for another, is a certain sign of developing healthy maturity.*

Once we realize we are individuals, and our actions with their joys and sorrows occur on a one-to-one basis, it is necessary to make the next jump in awareness. Although each of us is a solitary person, we live together in closely-related groups. These we label variously as "family," "peer group," and "society." Within these social groupings we must consider that our actions, or decisions to act, and their consequences, will affect other members of that society. It is for this reason that communities develop codes of behavior or laws governing what people may do. Often, these laws have application to sexual behavior.

Here we may logically reach a third generalization: Just as the laws of society affect the behavior of the individual members, so may the action of one member have far-reaching effects on his society. For example, in sexual behavior, a single act of intercourse by a VD carrier may enlarge the reservoir of infected people, further spreading gonorrhea or syphilis.

Irresponsibility in these areas of behavior has always perplexed me. We can cite cases of venereal disease involving a bank teller who is careful and responsible about the movement of thousands of dollars which daily pass through her hands; yet she knowingly spreads gonorrhea. Or the ambitious and outstanding student who takes pride in never cheating on exams, and who is thrilled and challenged by his studies; he, too, irresponsibly spreads VD. And there's the sailor who while at sea discharges technical and hazardous duties on which the lives of

117

many depend. Yet on shore—well, sailors (I was once one myself!) have a well-earned reputation for sexual irresponsibility and VD. Or the student nurse, or . . . On and on goes the catalogue of our societal schizophrenia, our split personality which enables us to behave morally at one moment and irresponsibly at another. We are now forced by circumstance to reappraise our actions in order to preserve our culture, if not our species.

In the sexual and reproductive sphere, Freud started us thinking about why we behave sexually as we do; Kinsey told us what we are doing; Masters and Johnson told us how to do it. *Now we must prepare ourselves to modify what we do and how we decide to do it, for our own good, and for the greater good of society.*

This challenge to individuals and to society to modify behavior seems insurmountable. "Boys will be boys" and "if she did it, she must pay the consequences" is as far as we have gotten in unnumbered thousands of years. Yet, I'm encouraged to think that it need not be this way, and I will now consider some of the aspects of our current techno-culture that makes me hopeful.

## THE SCHOOLS

Once a child begins to interact with the external or out-of-family society, as in church or school, the necessity for additional educational materials at appropriate levels becomes manifest. Sex education must continue in the schools, in order to supplement the groundwork begun at home, and to begin appropriate educational programs for those children whose parents have not been as positive about sex education. In the early childhood years, the information given should be simple and factual general material about sex and reproduction. In the preadolescent

118

years, both boys and girls should learn about the adolescent phase of growth in both sexes. Girls need to know what is going to happen to boys: hair growth, deepening of voice, sexual awakening, and masturbation. Boys need to know what will happen to girls: menstruation, breast and hip development, delayed sexual awakening, less frequent masturbation. This cross-sexual education is a must, since it leads to healthier knowledge around which adult decision-making processes may grow and develop.

Once adolescence settles down, the educational program should expand to include factual material about marriage, the family, and child rearing. Included must be material covering problematic behavior, including out-of-wedlock pregnancy, homosexuality, abortion, drugs, and venereal diseases. The process by which we make decisions is another important topic; this subject, which also involves moral and ethical values, is often effectively discussed in small groups where questions are more easily asked and answered. Programs may be carried out under the supervision of churches and youth groups in your local community, as some questions involving ethical and moral behavior are more comfortably discussed there. Of course, sex education is difficult in a diverse society but nonetheless, it *must* be provided.

I have personally participated in sex education programs in local churches, involving both parents and their sons and daughters, and feel such an experience is useful to bring specific knowledge and viewpoints into the religious community. It is an obligation that both the churches and skilled professionals like myself must willingly undertake. The primary target, however, should still be the schools, since this is the principal place where *all* young people at risk for sexual and VD problems gather.

By exposing young people to an ongoing, long-term sex education program, utilizing the resources of family,

119

physicians, trained professionals, religious institutions, and schools, I believe larger proportions of youth will reach maturity well able to understand the physical and emotional forces that drive them. This knowledge will help guide them to intelligent, informed, and responsible decisions regarding their sexual activities. In this context, I cannot help but feel that prevention of VD will be the logical end result when an informed human being lives among peers with similar views. I do not imply this will come about by persuading the young to not have intercourse. I do not believe sexual abstinence should be either the primary objective of sex education, or the major means of assaying the effectiveness of sex education programs. But, if young people can see that intelligent use of their natures is a reasonable choice open to them, prevention of VD will become a frame of mind for all, rather than an unheard plaintive cry from the Department of Public Health.

## THE MEDIA

It is also time for our society to come to grips with the media that surround and bombard us with messages of all sorts. Regarding sex, these communications are usually pleasure-seeking and irresponsible, with a commercial overtone. Sex is used to sell anything and everything, from underwear to automobiles. Since this message is known to be effective, is it not possible to use the tremendous teaching potential of the media for some meaningful purpose?

There are glimmerings that this might be gradually taking place; the recent decision to ban all cigarette advertising from television and radio is a case in point. It implies a future concern for health that might spill over from lung cancer and heart disease into human sexuality. One of the popular "MD" television programs had an episode concerned with VD, giving it frank and accurate treatment.

Local audiences demonstrate increasing interest and receptivity to educational programs on these topics. Several other physicians and I recently participated in an informative television panel discussion on VD which was remarkably well received in our community. Out of concern for the public interest, both television stations and interested and skilled professionals must provide more of this kind of programming.

The radio talk-master is another person who can help. I have had the pleasure to be both a direct participant and a "hot line" consultant to Boston radio programs discussing sex education, VD, birth control, and abortion. One good television or radio program of this sort can reach more people in one showing than I could professionally contact in a lifetime on the lecture circuit, in the church youth group or in my office.

I foresee the day when the "sexpert" participates in an ongoing talk show in the same manner that some local stations have used theologians, psychologists, and sports figures to provide their special expertise; it will be a welcome development. *The day will come when all divisions of the media live up to their potential for disseminating useful information about sexuality, instead of debasing sex as a commercial instrument. Our communications technology will truly have come of age.*

## THE OPPOSITION

Whenever a program of home and public education about human sexuality, its hazards as well as its joys, is

121

proposed, there must be some consideration of the opposition which will be encountered. More or less organized groups of parents that fear this kind of effort are found everywhere, but I think their objections can all be reasonably met. Here are their five major points, and my responses to them.

ONE. "Sex education belongs in the home, not in the schools."

I agree that it does belong in the home, and have hopes that more and more families will realize this and prepare themselves to carry out programs with their children. But the vast majority of homes do little or nothing, or they are actively negative. Surprisingly often, those parents who do the least, or are the most negative, are the very ones who oppose sex education in the schools. Obviously, the emergency nature of the current situation demands that *both* homes and schools become involved, since each has an important role in the appropriate sex education of young people. The school program can often provide a relaxed atmosphere for the child's exploration of material that would be threatening at home, and could also provide a springboard for more thorough and informative home discussions.

TWO. "What is to be taught?"

This, of course, is a big factor in any program. Well-thought-out curricular materials are available from many sources, some in your own local area. Others are obtainable from national agencies specializing in the provision of educational and teaching material for use in these subjects. The community itself needs an important voice when choosing the subject matter in order to involve its members with the problems of sex and venereal disease. The schools and churches should make use of local professional people in their programs. It must be clear to all, moreover, that there will be no hedging of facts, and that there will be an emphasis on fostering intelligent, informed and responsible decision-making by each student. Parents must be notified in advance of the curricular content and given the opportunity to discuss it. All should be aware that diverse moral and ethical views will be presented.

THREE. "Who is going to teach sex education?"

Once again, this is a valid point. A school system should give highest priority to finding within the system, or recruiting from outside, those individuals who are stable, capable, and interested in teaching young people about human sexuality. Once selected, they can be further educated for the job that the schools and parents need them to do. There are now in existence summer courses specifically designed for training in sex education. I think carefully chosen instructors who are appropriately trained can satisfy the most reluctant parent. Parents can be assured that the teacher's credentials are better than those of the untrained coach or the school nurse, and certainly better than those of curious but ignorant peers in back-alley discussion groups.

FOUR. "Why should we bother with sex education in the schools—my children don't need it, since I've given them all they need at home." Or: "Why are you so concerned about sex education? I can teach my children all they need to know about sex in half an hour."

This in some ways is the hardest position to change, since these people honestly believe what they are saying. Unfortunately it just isn't true, especially within the context of the current youth culture. Quite often this parent is totally unaware of what his own children are doing,

123

even when they have gotten into trouble. In many cases that I have seen, the child in trouble conceals his or her situation, be it pregnancy, VD, or anxiety-producing sexual activity, from the parent, because the problem cannot be handled within the family. These parents should know the full extent of what is happening in the community through their local publications. For parents and children alike, learning about sexual activity, and coming to grips with it, is a lifelong process—not a one-shot affair.

There's no person active in the field of human sexuality, including myself, who considers he knows all there is to know. We are all still learning. If this is true of gynecologists, psychologists, and sex educators, it is likely that the average young person can also learn something of use and value to him at school, regardless of how much he has been taught at home.

FIVE. "Sex education programs are part of a great communist conspiracy to destroy the morals of the young."

Surprisingly, this viewpoint has some strong and effective adherents; in certain parts of the country it has set back the progress of enlightened sex education by a matter of years. It is fostered by those who believe that teaching sex encourages promiscuity and irresponsibility. Since it is human and convenient to blame others for problems some of us cannot handle, it is easy to shift guilt, as in this case to a communist conspiracy.

There is no truth in this accusation. I personally feel it is ridiculous and not worthy of further comment.

If one thinks carefully and rationally, it becomes obvious that in recent years the moral values of American young have not come from sex education, but have been acquired from the wrong sources, i.e., the media, commercial interests, and ignorant and wrongly motivated adults and peers. Carrying this clear, careful, and rational thinking a few steps further brings you to the inevitable conclusion that the time has come to bring the teaching of human sexuality up to date, utilizing all the knowledge we presently possess and the newest and best of our teaching methods. Any other consideration is a cop out. Your failure to do your part is at the expense of your children, my children, and yourself.

## SIX THOUGHTS FOR VD PREVENTION

1. Adults, young people, and society in general must accept that we have a medical and social problem of major dimensions. Venereal diseases have now become the most common communicable infections in the country.
2. Parents and other adults need to create and provide for the young an appropriate education that gives them facts about sexuality, reproduction, venereal diseases, and drugs. Homes, schools, and religious institutions should all participate.
3. Learning to make responsible decisions is of equal importance to men, women, and children. Responsible decisions lead to appropriate actions.
4. The importance of caring for each individual as a person, whether it be self or another person, must be taught and lived by adults. Young people will then learn both by precept and example.
5. Each of us must realize that in the final analysis, the sexual experience involves only two persons, eyeball to eyeball, and body to body. Within that personal context, we must care for one another, and make decisions that consider consequences as parts of actions taken.
6. *VD IS PREVENTED BY PEOPLE.*

125

I hope that you, your parents, and your girl friends and boyfriends will read and reread the last several chapters, and use them or any other parts of the book as bases for discussion. You may disagree with my ideas, which is O.K. by me. None of you, however, can deny any longer the truth about what's happening "out there." You must act, or the situation cannot improve.

## CHAPTER 15

## TEEN-AGE RAP SESSION

Much of my thinking about human sexuality, reproduction, and the current problem of venereal disease has grown from my interactions with young people. My home church in Weston, St. Peter's Episcopal Church, for five years has been a frequent location for rap sessions. The questions and answers presented here came out of a series of discussions this winter, and I am grateful to the young people for their participation, and for permitting their pictures to be taken at one evening's rap. I think the material that follows shows most forcefully what can and needs to be done.

### FIFTEEN QUESTIONS AND ANSWERS ABOUT VD

1. *Why are there venereal diseases anyway?*
   Venereal diseases represent special kinds of bacterial or virus-like infections that have counterparts in all of the body's organ systems. The unique aspects of the sexual and reproductive relationship allow for their passage from one person to another. We assume they have existed since very ancient times, as have most diseases.

127

2. *How are venereal diseases contracted?*
These diseases are contracted through intimate touching of the moist surfaces of the body, especially the genitals. Rarely, the mouth or the rectum are the original site of infection.

3. *How many venereal diseases are there?*
Syphilis and gonorrhea make up ninety-five percent of all cases in the United States. Gonorrhea is about twenty times as prevalent as syphilis. The less common diseases include chancroid, lymphogranuloma venereum, and granuloma inguinale. There also are minor sexually transmitted conditions, such as trichomonas vaginitis, monilia, and crab lice.

4. *Can you catch venereal diseases from a toilet seat or dirty bathtub?*
This is a common excuse, but rarely if ever true. The organisms are so sensitive to temperature changes and drying that they quickly die when out of contact with the body. Infrequently, nurses or doctors may develop syphilis if they cut or stick themselves during surgery in a syphilitic patient.

5. *How do you know if you have VD?*
The first symptoms often pass unnoticed. There may be a small sore or ulcer if it is syphilis, or a "drip" from the urethra if it is gonorrhea. Painful and frequent urination may be early signs of gonorrhea.

6. *Will you always have symptoms if you have VD?*
No. Particularly in women, a symptomless carrier-state for gonorrhea exists. A woman may spread the disease for an indefinite period before she develops any sign of infection.

7. *Can you tell if your partner has VD?*
Generally not. The early signs may be missed, and he or she may either be a carrier or in an inactive stage.

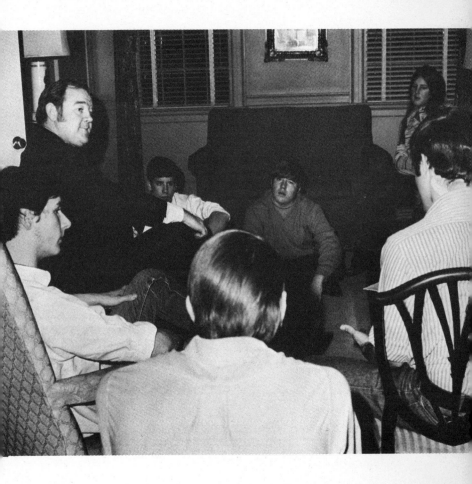

8. *How long does it take to cure VD?*
Since the development of antibiotics such as penicillin, both syphilis and gonorrhea are effectively treated in a few days' time. However, in all cases, proper follow-up to insure cure is necessary.

9. *Where can I go to get treatment if I suspect that I have VD?*
You should go to your doctor, or to the nearest clinic or hospital with facilities for diagnosing and treating VD. You should not attempt self-treatment or take folk remedies. You should be frank with your doctor, and be ready to list contacts so that they, too, can be effectively treated.

10. *Can VD affect male and female fertility?*
Yes, in both sexes. Repeated or neglected cases, particularly of gonorrhea, can cause sterility by damaging the passageways that carry sperm or eggs. We are now not far from having a sterile generation of young people because so many have been infected with gonorrhea.

11. *Can VD be transmitted to an unborn child?*
Yes, in two ways. Syphilis can be passed through the blood stream to the baby growing in the womb, where it may cause severe damage and even stillbirth. Gonorrhea can be given to a baby at the time of birth, and blindness may result.

12. *Do animals have venereal diseases?*
Yes, at least as far as dogs are concerned. It is known that they may have several sexually-spread diseases similar to gonorrhea and syphilis. Human and canine diseases are not interchangeable, and there is no known animal reservoir for the human venereal diseases.

13. *Can VD be prevented?*
Yes. The guidelines for venereal disease prevention include learning to be responsible and thoughtful about sexual activity. *We should be willing to defer intercourse in any relationship un-*

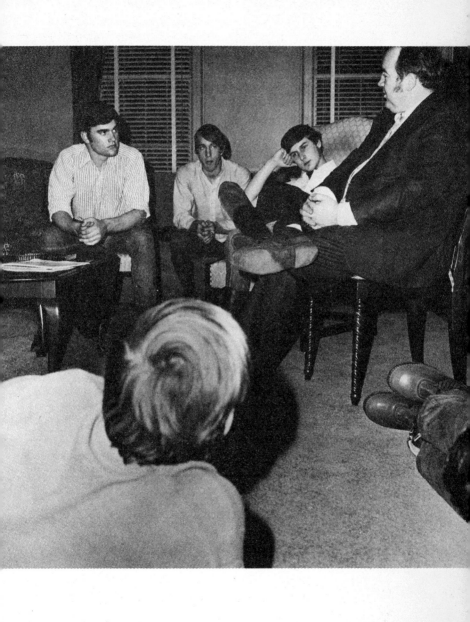

*til we are truly prepared to use the sexual side of our nature in a healthy and fulfilling way with our partner, not just for casual fun.* We must be frank and careful with each other and willing to do all we can to prevent VD's and to treat them rapidly when they occur. There is too much at stake for us to be irresponsible.

14. *If I had VD when I was young, will anyone ever know later?*

If you were wise as well as fortunate, and were treated early and effectively, unless you reveal your history there is no way anyone can ever know. However, the longer VD is untreated the more evidence it will leave behind, including sterility or actual tissue damage. So many people in the future will have had VD that you must be prepared either to frankly reveal your own or compassionately understand your partner's past problems.

15. *Are venereal diseases really more common than they used to be?*

Yes, without doubt. There have been times in the past when they occurred frequently, but now they are increasing rapidly and uncontrollably all over the world, in every segment and level of society.

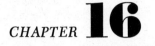

## VENEREAL DISEASE:
## AN INSTANT REPLAY

Some of the chapters in this book may seem more technical than they should be, and some may seem longer than they should be. For those of you who couldn't stay with it page by page, and for those of you who are practicing your rapid-reading techniques, the following summary of VD is provided. You are all invited to browse and study elsewhere in the book at your leisure; hopefully, I can entice you into doing just that. The summary is divided into three parts: Facts, Viewpoints, and Challenges.

### FACTS

1. Venereal diseases exist. They are spread through sexual intercourse. Doorknobs, bathtubs, and toilet seats are not involved.
2. The major VD's are syphilis and gonorrhea. Over ninety-five percent of all serious venereal infections in the United States are due to these two diseases.
3. Once you are infected, syphilis spreads throughout the body, and can affect your unborn child. It can kill you, or maim you for life.
4. Gonorrhea is usually a localized genital infection.

133

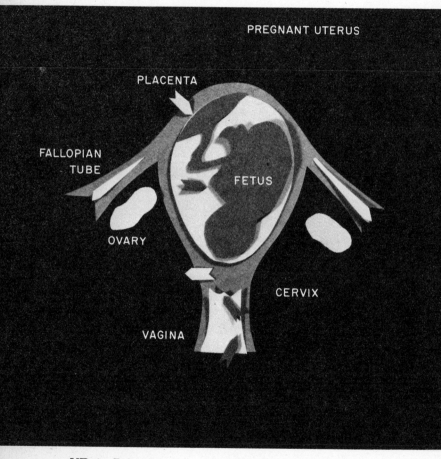

## VD in Pregnancy

The point of infection is the vagina or cervix. The diseases may spread through the blood or lymph vessels, but only syphilis can cross the placenta to the baby.

It can often cause sterility. It can also cause blindness in newborn babies.

5. Women are more likely to have VD without knowing it than men, and therefore are apt to spread disease to many contacts before being treated.

6. VD is curable with antibiotics. Penicillin is the best choice for syphilis and gonorrhea, although others are effective.

7. The longer VD's are untreated, the more damage they do. Immunity is not acquired by infection.

8. VD is increasing faster in teen-agers than in any other age group. Over five hundred thousand teen-agers will contract gonorrhea or syphilis in the United States in 1971. Nearly one million five hundred thousand total cases will be seen.

9. VD remains a problem in older people and crosses all socioeconomic barriers. No group is exempt from risk.

10. There are minor sexually transmitted conditions which mimic VD, and cause unwarranted distress.

11. Proven VD should be reported to your local Department of Public Health for proper contact tracing, and for the prevention of further spread.

## VIEWPOINTS

1. The current epidemic of VD is related to the increased casualness of sexual relationships, particularly in young people, and to ignorant or irresponsible attitudes toward infection and its treatment.

2. The epidemic is further related to affluence, to the commercialization and dehumanization of sex, and to peer-group pressures leading to conformity in seeking sexual experience and gratification.

3. It is better to prevent VD than it is to treat it, though treatment is obviously important.

135

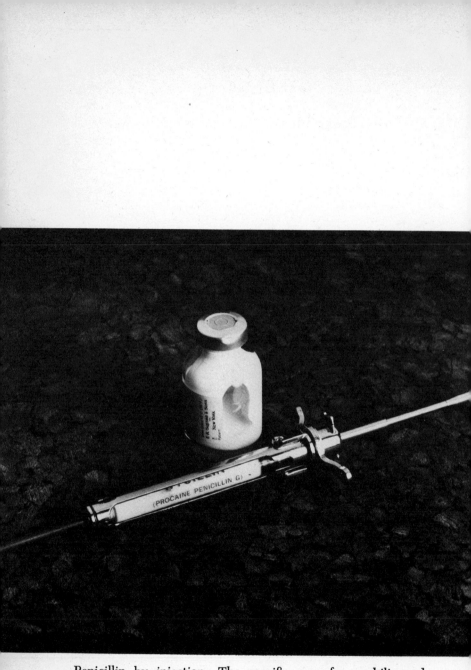

Penicillin by injection: The specific cure for syphilis and gonorrhea in most cases. See your doctor for the right dose.

4. Prevention of VD must be fostered by appropriate sex education in the homes, schools, and churches. The vast capacity of the mass media for education and dissemination of factual materials and viewpoints should be exploited.

5. A person can often prevent VD by waiting a few weeks before beginning a new sexual relationship, staying with one partner, using mechanical or chemical protection whenever possible, and observing good personal hygiene. Do not have intercourse if you have symptoms of VD. *When in doubt observe the rule: No one ever died from not having intercourse.*

6. VD must be treated as soon as possible, and careful follow-up observed to insure complete cure.

## CHALLENGES

1. Each person is challenged by his own sexual needs and desires, to use them responsibly and wisely, to the harm of no one.

2. Each family is challenged to provide a loving and wholesome atmosphere for the nurture of children in such a way that meaningful and appropriate knowledge about human sexuality, including VD, is imparted. The children in turn must learn to make responsible decisions for action in these important areas.

3. The schools and churches are challenged to provide additional appropriate information to complement that given in the home, so that young people may have the possibility of arriving at maturity sensibly and responsibly, without making blunders through ignorance.

4. The fabric of our entire society is challenged by the current epidemic of diseases of ancient lineage, which occur ever increasingly in spite of our

modern medical knowledge and our sophistication about sex. Are we to be a nation of people brought to its knees by incredible mass irresponsibility and ignorance, or will we be able to stand tall and build a more healthy and safe society for ourselves and for our children?

Each of these points of summation can become a focus for discussion with further amplification using what I have written elsewhere in the text. I hope you have found the book informative and useful. Please remember that it comes from someone who cares a lot about the people whom he has had the privilege and pleasure of having as patients, and who would like to see it different and better —for his kids and their friends, now and in the years to come.

# APPENDIX

How to get information on VD clinics and treatment when you are in trouble:

1. Department of Public Health in your state—look for section on communicable diseases or VD.
2. Call your city hospital VD department.
3. Hospital telephone operators will have information on VD clinics in any general hospital.
4. Check your nearest sex, drug, and VD "Hot Line" —see your college or school paper for these local numbers. Often "Hot Lines" are listed in underground newspapers.
5. Contact or visit a "Free Clinic" (like the MGH Medivan) in your vicinity.
6. If you have a regular doctor, he can be a source of information as well as treatment.
7. Military people should make their VD problem known early at sick call and get prompt treatment.
8. If you are in school or college your health clinic can be used if you wish; otherwise, seek care through an outside source.
9. A registered pharmacist in your local drugstore will know where to refer you for VD information and treatment.

10. If you suspect that you have VD while traveling abroad, the following contacts may be helpful:
    (A.) American Express Office
    (B.) The nearest American Embassy or Consulate
11. Remember that self-treatment is dangerous and ineffective. You owe too much to yourself to risk poor medical attention.
12. For a comprehensive list of places where VD assistance may be obtained all over the United States, you can write to:

> U.S. Department of Health,
> Education and Welfare
> Public Health Service
> Communicable Disease Center
> Venereal Disease Branch
> Atlanta, Georgia, 30333

The book you will receive is entitled:
*Telephone Guide for Rapid Transmission of Venereal Disease Epidemiologic Information.*

If you're in trouble and near any of these places, then call:

| City | Phone # |
|---|---|
| Atlanta, Georgia | (404)656-4937 |
| Augusta, Maine | (207)289-1110 |
| Austin, Texas | (512)454-3781 |
| Baltimore, Maryland | (301)383-2644 |
| Berkeley, California (also includes San Francisco) | (415)843-7900 |
| Boston, Massachusetts | (617)727-2681 |
| Chicago, Illinois | (312)793-2793 |
| Columbus, Ohio | (614)461-7367 |
| Denver, Colorado | (303)388-6111 |
| Detroit, Michigan | (313)872-1540 |
| Frankfort, Kentucky | (502)564-4935 |
| Harrisburg, Pennsylvania | (717)787-8842 |
| Hartford, Connecticut | (203)566-4140 |

| *City* | *Phone #* |
|---|---|
| Honolulu, Hawaii | (808)548-2211 |
| Indianapolis, Indiana | (317)633-6310 |
| Jackson, Mississippi | (904)354-3961 |
| Jefferson City, Missouri | (314)635-4111 |
| Juneau, Alaska | (907)586-5301 |
| (Community Health) | (907)586-5407 |
| Los Angeles, California | (213)620-2900 |
| Minneapolis, Minnesota | (612)378-1150 |
| Montgomery, Alabama | (205)269-7606 |
| Nashville, Tennessee | (615)741-3614 |
| New Orleans, Louisiana | (504)527-5816 |
| New York City, New York | (212)971-5647 |
| Oklahoma City, Oklahoma . | (405)427-6561 |
| Olympia, Washington | (206)753-5900 |
| Phoenix, Arizona | (602)271-4521 |
| Philadelphia, Pennsylvania | (215)238-7703 |
| Raleigh, North Carolina | (919)829-3419 |
| Richmond, Virginia | (703)770-6265 |
| San Diego, California | (714)232-4361 |
| San Francisco, California (also includes Berkeley, California) | (415)843-7900 |
| Santa Fe, New Mexico | (505)827-2107 |
| Trenton, New Jersey | (609)292-4027 |
| Washington, D.C. | (202)655-4000 |

## IN CANADA

| | |
|---|---|
| Edmonton, Alberta | (403)422-6596 |
| Vancouver, British Columbia | (604)874-2331 |
| Winnipeg, Manitoba | (204)946-7746 |
| Fredericton, New Brunswick | (506)475-7711 |
| St. Johns, Newfoundland | (709)726-2610 |
| Halifax, Nova Scotia | (902)424-4431 |
| Toronto, Ontario | (416)365-4058 |
| Charlottetown, Prince Edward Island | (902)892-3481 |
| Quebec City, Quebec | (418)643-6430 |
| Regina, Saskatchewan | (306)523-0661 |

# GLOSSARY

Abortion: Early termination of pregnancy, usually during the first three months. Abortions may be spontaneous or induced.

Aneurysm: A swelling or dilatation of a major blood vessel (sometimes due to syphilis in its later stages).

Antibiotic: A chemical that destroys or stops the growth of bacteria. Penicillin, tetracycline, and streptomycin are common ones.

Anus: External opening from the rectum.

Asymptomatic: Without signs or symptoms; that stage of a disease when there are no symptoms.

Birth-Control Pills: Any of several varieties of orally effective sex hormone preparations; they control fertility by suppressing ovulation.

Carrier: A person who transmits diseases without having symptoms. The carrier stage of VD is usually of limited duration.

Cervix: The lower end of the uterus. Sperm must pass through the cervix in order to fertilize an egg, and initiate pregnancy.

Chancre: The primary ulcer or lesion of syphilis. It can be painless and unnoticed. Chancres may appear anywhere on the body, wherever the initial infection occurs.

Chancroid: A venereal disease caused by Ducrey's bacillus. It produces severe genital ulceration, swelling, and drainage of lymph nodes. More common in the tropics.

Clap: Slang term; gonorrhea.

Coitus Interruptus: Birth-control method where the penis is withdrawn from the vagina at the time of ejaculation. Not effective in preventing pregnancy.

Condom: Mechanical method of birth control using a rubber or skin-like sheath covering the penis; it is moderately effective.

Congenital Syphilis: Syphilis passed across the placenta from the mother to the fetus. If the child is born alive, malformed teeth and bones and mental retardation are common.

Crabs: An infestation of genital skin with the pubic louse, a parasitic insect; it is spread through body contact or dirty clothing.

Dark-field Preparation: A study for syphilis spirochetes; a slide containing a wet smear taken directly from a chancre and studied under a microscope using special lighting.

Diaphragm: Mechanical birth-control device; a disc-like rubber membrane placed deep within the vagina to prevent sperm from reaching the cervix. It is used with contraceptive jelly and quite effective if properly inserted.

Douche: To wash the vagina with a cleansing or medicated solution.

"Drip": Pus-like exudate from urethra of persons with gonorrhea; slang for gonorrhea.

Egg: Germ cell of the female, also called an ovum. Usually one is released each month by a process known as ovulation.

Extended Family: The nuclear family (parents and children) plus all other relatives, grandparents, cousins, etc.

Fallopian Tubes: Tubular passageways that carry the egg from ovary to uterus after ovulation. These tubes are

143

often irreparably damaged by gonorrheal infection, causing sterility.

Fertility: The ability to conceive and bear children. Loss of this capacity is known as infertility or sterility.

Fetus: The unborn child after the third month of pregnancy.

"French Pox": Old term for syphilis, used by the English.

G.C.: Slang term for gonorrhea.

Generation Gap: The differences in experiences and viewpoints of parents and their children. It always exists, is especially obvious at present due to the rapid social changes of the last decades, including wars and the proliferation of mass media.

Genitals: Primary sexual organs. Male genitals are the penis and testicles; female genitals are the vulva, vagina, uterus, tubes, and ovaries.

Gonorrhea: Most common venereal disease in the United States. It is caused by the bacteria, *Neisseria gonorrhoeae* and often causes local inflammation in the genital tract. It can spread to the rest of the body and is a cause of blindness in newborns. Also called clap, the "drip," or G.C.

Gram Stain: Special staining technique to identify gonorrheal organisms under a microscope.

Granuloma Inguinale: A less common venereal disease caused by bacteria. Severe ulceration of genitals and local tissues occur. Seen mostly in the tropics, but also in southern U.S.A.

Gumma: An abscess seen late in a syphilitic infection. It can occur in and destroy any organ of the body.

"Hang-up": A mental block or inhibition. To be inhibited is to be "hung up."

Herpes Progenitalis: Virus infection of genitals which may cause ulceration of the penis or labia minora. It is not serious, but is easily mistaken for syphilis.

Herxheimer Reaction: A temporary rash and fever which may occur when a patient is first treated for syphilis with penicillin.

144

Hymen: Small fold of mucous membrane encircling the opening to the vagina. An intact hymen is considered a sign of virginity.

Hysterectomy: Surgical removal of the uterus; often the fallopian tubes and ovaries are removed as well.

Intercourse: The act of love, or coitus; placement of the erect penis within the vagina. This is the most common way to transmit a venereal disease.

Intrauterine: Inside the cavity of the uterus.

Intrauterine Contraceptive Devices (IUD): Mechanical devices placed inside the uterus by a physician in order to prevent pregnancy.

Lues: A synonym for syphilis.

Lymphogranuloma Venereum: A venereal disease caused by a virus-like organism. It is seen mostly in the tropics and causes ulceration of the genitals and surrounding tissues.

Menstruation: The monthly flow of blood from the womb of women during the childbearing years.

Monilia (*Candida albicans*): An irritating yeast infection, causing itching, redness, and swelling of the genitals. It can affect both sexes.

Mucous Membrane: Moist body coverings, as in the mouth, rectum, vagina, and urethra.

Neonatal: The first few days of newborn life.

Neurosyphilis: Late or tertiary syphilis affecting the brain or spinal cord. It may cause paralysis, blindness, deafness, and insanity.

Nonspecific Urethritis: Obscure group of nongonococcal infections of uncertain etiology, affecting both sexes.

Nuclear Family: The immediate family consisting of father, mother, and children, without other relatives in the household.

Ophthalmia Neonatorum: Irritation and inflammation of the eyes in newborns, usually caused by congenital gonorrheal infection. Blindness may result.

Ovaries: Two round pelvic glands, one on either side of the uterus. They hold many eggs in the mature female and usually release one each month in order that pregnancy may occur. Ovaries provide hormonal mechanisms which govern the menstrual cycles and support early pregnancy.

Ovulation: The production of an egg by the ovary.

Pandemic: Nationwide spread of any disease, infecting vast numbers of people, as in an epidemic, but covering a broader area.

Pelvic Inflammatory Disease (P.I.D.): Advanced state of gonorrhea or other pelvic infection in the female. The uterus, tubes, and ovaries are inflamed and may be permanently damaged causing sterility.

Penis: External male sexual organ. It functions as the urinary outlet, ejaculates sperm when erect and sexually stimulated.

Peritonitis: An infection or inflammation of the abdominal cavity.

Placenta: The spongy vascular organ that allows the interchange of oxygen, nutrients, and waste materials between the mother and her unborn baby. It is also known as the "afterbirth."

Pregnancy: The duration of intrauterine growth and development for each baby. It begins with implantation and ends at birth.

Prophylaxis: A prevention or protection, usually against diseases. Medicines offer protection against disease, while birth-control devices are prophylaxis against pregnancy or VD.

Prostate Gland: Gland surrounding the male urethra at the base of the bladder. It provides secretions for sperm transport during ejaculation. If infected by gonorrhea, male sterility may result.

Puerperal Sepsis: Infection of the pelvic organs of a woman following the delivery of a baby; "childbed fever."

Reproduction: The processes of conception, pregnancy, and birth.

Scabies: Infestation with an insect (mite) which burrows

146

under the skin, causing an itchy rash. It is spread by body contact.

Sex Education: The teaching of sexuality and reproduction, primarily to young people. In this book. the term is used with a broad interpretation.

Stillbirth: The birth of a dead fetus, usually meaning a baby sufficiently developed to have survived otherwise.

Syphilis: A venereal disease caused by a bacterium, the spiral-shaped spirochete, *Treponema pallidum*. It may spread to any part of the body, including the brain, and can be fatal. Syphilis can harm unborn babies.

Tabes Dorsalis: Paralysis; a form of neurosyphilis.

Testicles: The two sperm-cell producing organs of the male. They are carried in a sac-like structure, the scrotum, hanging below the penis.

Trichomonas Vaginitis: Vaginal infection caused by a protozoal parasite, *Trichomonas vaginalis*. It produces an irritating discharge, and can be carried by a male partner, who usually has no symptoms.

Urethra: Passageway through which urine passes from the urinary bladder to the outside of the body. In the male, it also functions to carry sperm. In both sexes, it can become inflamed from a gonorrheal infection, or be the site of a syphilitic chancre.

Uterus: Womb; a pear-shaped muscular internal female sex organ which provides a place for the development of the fetus. In its nonpregnant state, it sheds its lining during menstruation.

Vagina: The female pelvic passageway from the outside of the body to the womb. During intercourse it receives the erect penis. It is the birth canal at the time of delivery.

Venereal Diseases: Any of a number of diseases spread primarily through sexual contact. Included are syphilis, gonorrhea, and several minor diseases.

Venereal Warts: Warty growths on the genitals, caused by

a viral infection. Often seen with other inflammatory conditions of the vagina.

Vulva: External female genitals. Its major structures are the hair-bearing labia majora, the moist labia minora, the clitoris, and the perineum.

Wassermann Test: Blood test to determine the presence of syphilis. The Hinton test is similar.

Yaws, Pinta, Bejel: Nonvenereal treponemal or spirochetal diseases seen in the tropics.